Brain Training Mastery

Advanced Learning Strategies to Improve and Expand Memory Concentration and Be More Focalized

Robert Olson

Text Copyright © [Robert Olsonl]

All rights reserved. No part of this guide may be reproduced in any form without permission in writing from the publisher except in the case of brief quotations embodied in critical articles or reviews.

Legal & Disclaimer
The information contained in this book and its contents is not designed to replace or take the place of any form of medical or professional advice; and is not meant to replace the need for independent medical, financial, legal or other professional advice or services, as may be required. The content and information in this book has been provided for educational and entertainment purposes only.
The content and information contained in this book has been compiled from sources deemed reliable, and it is accurate to the best of the Author's knowledge, information and belief. However, the Author cannot guarantee its accuracy and validity and cannot be held liable for any errors and/or omissions. Further, changes are periodically made to this book as and when needed. Where appropriate and/or necessary, you must consult a professional (including but not limited to your doctor, attorney, financial advisor or such other professional advisor) before using any of the suggested remedies, techniques, or information in this book.
Upon using the contents and information contained in this book, you agree to hold harmless the Author from and against any damages, costs, and expenses, including any legal fees potentially resulting from the application of any of the information provided by this book. This disclaimer applies to any loss, damages or injury caused by the use and application, whether directly or indirectly, of any advice or information presented, whether for breach of contract, tort, negligence, personal injury, criminal intent, or under any other cause of action.
You agree to accept all risks of using the information presented inside this book.
You agree that by continuing to read this book, where appropriate and/or necessary, you shall consult a professional (including but not limited to your doctor, attorney, or financial advisor or such other advisor as needed) before using any of the suggested remedies, techniques, or information in this book.

Table of Contents

TABLE OF CONTENTS

INTRODUCTION

CHAPTER 1: THE BRAIN

The Nervous System

The Brain's Central Role

The Left vs. the Right

Emotions and the Brain

Stress and the Brain

The Importance of Sleep

CHAPTER 2: CONCENTRATION

What is Concentration?

The Importance of Concentration

Improving Concentration

Concentration, Learning, and Forgetting

The Repetition Method

CHAPTER 3: ASSOCIATION

Learning by Association

How Association Works

Using Association

Association Through Sounds

Association by Song

CHAPTER 4: CONNECTIONS

Making Connections

Boosting Focus with Connections

Using Connections

Making Connections in Practice

CHAPTER 5: PHOTOGRAPHIC MEMORY

What is Photographic Memory?

Developing a Photographic Memory

How Photographic Memory Boosts Focus

The Military Method for Photographic Memory

Discovering Mind Maps

How Mind Maps Work

Using Mind Maps

CHAPTER 7: THE BODY AND REMEMBERING

The Body and Memory

The Senses and Memory

Using the Body and Memory

Clenching Fists to Concentrate and Remember

Moving Eyes From Side to Side to Improve Learning

Practical Exercises to Train the Brain
  Remembering Names and Faces
  Remind yourself of your motivator
  If you know that this name and face is important, remind yourself of what is on the hook if you fail to remember it. Is this the name of your new boss or the person that interviewed you? Is it the name of someone who will be relevant to you later on?
  Remembering Numbers and Data
  Consider the number as if it were being typed on a number pad
  Remembering Directions
  Associate an image with left and right
  Repeat them back
  Turn it into a story
  Create landmarks and associations
  Remembering Shopping Lists
  Write your list in a silly font
  Use a memory palace
  Create nonsense acronyms
  If, at the end of the day, what you need is memorable, what is more memorable than something that sounds ridiculous? If you have children, you may be able to turn it into a game—who can make the most ridiculous sounding acronym with the shopping list to make sure that it is memorable? Your children's abilities may surprise you.
  Using Creativity
  Repeating things back to yourself—but in different words
  Let your imagination run free
  Calculation
  Replacing subtracting with addition
  Multiply in parts instead of as a whole
  Multiplying by 4 or 8 just requires you to double numbers
  Speed Reading
  The pointer method
  The track and pace method
  The scanning method
  Brain Food
  Physical Exercises for the Brain

CONCLUSION

Introduction

Congratulations on purchasing *Brain Training Mastery,* and thank you for doing so.

Your brain controls everything. Like a well-oiled machine, it is responsible for everything, from keeping you alive to help you think critically about a situation in order to solve problems. It allows you to read, remember a phone number, and do anything else that you need to get done throughout your day. Your brain, then, is the pinnacle of everything that is you. Without it, you could not live. Without it, you could not think. This means that your brain's health and strength is absolutely essential if you wish to be a happy and healthy person.

Just as you can train and strengthen other body parts as well, you can also make it a point to train and strengthen your brain. In fact, doing so can dramatically increase your own cognitive abilities. Even if you have found that you have always struggled to commit things to memory or to keep track of everything you need to do in your day-to-day life, you can learn to do better. This is the sole purpose of brain training.

Through training your brain, you can develop the cognitive abilities that you thought you would never be able to claim.

You can ensure that you can, in fact, remember lists of groceries without having to write them down. You can become so much more efficient as you go through your day, not having to waste time trying to take notes and ensure that you can remember things. Instead, you will be able to rely on several tactics to make mental notes, strengthening your mind, and teaching yourself to be able to remember almost automatically.

Over time, these methods will become automatic.

This book will teach you to do just that. In reading this book, you will learn all about how the brain works and how to begin using the brain's natural strengths to yourself. You will be guided through several different techniques and tools that you can use to strengthen your own mind, ranging from concentration to using the body as a memory aid.

Finally, you'll be guided through practical exercises that will help you in a wide range of contexts that you are likely to run into on a regular basis. You will learn how to remember names, faces, data, directions, shopping lists, and more. You will also be given a list of exercises and foods to eat in order to make sure that your body is in the optimal condition to be used.

After all, no matter how much training you do, you still need to ensure that your body and brain have the right tools to thrive.

Upon finishing up with this book, you will have the tools you need. Having those tools means that you will be able to take control of your life. You will be able to ensure that you are always working to your fullest potential.

There are plenty of books on this subject on the market, thanks again for choosing this one! Every effort was made to ensure it is full of as much useful information as possible; please enjoy!

Chapter 1: The Brain

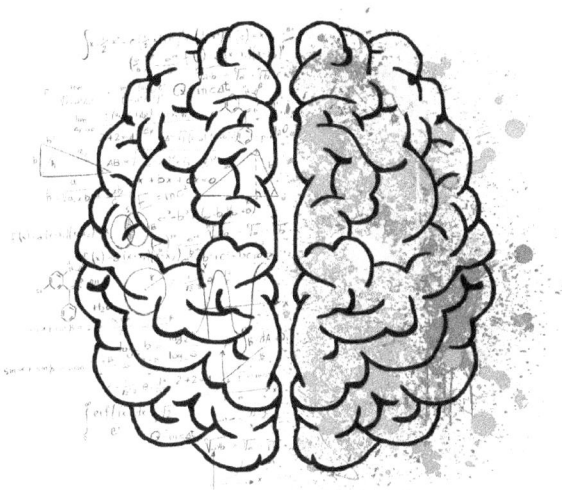

Your body is made up of a wide range of parts.

Your heart keeps blood pumping around your body. Your lungs keep your blood oxygenated. Your muscles allow you to move, and your digestive tracts allow you to take in all of the nutrients that you need in order to be healthy. Above it all, however, is the brain.

The brain is the main powerhouse behind the entire body, without the brain, the body cannot function.

Think of a computer for a moment.

When you are using your computer, several different components are working together. There is the processor, which does all of the thinking, and the power supply, which provides the power. Then, there are all sorts of other connections that run and work together, allowing you to work.

Your brain is like the processor, it is the part of your brain that actively pieces together all input and output, figuring out how to respond and acting accordingly.
Your brain is responsible for it all.
Through a series of nerves, known as both afferent and efferent, impulses are translated and sent either to the brain or to the body, commanding the body what to do next.

Within this chapter, we will delve into the brain. We will discuss how to best understand the nervous system, what the brain does, emotions, stress, and how it relates to the brain, and the importance of sleep.
In reading through this chapter, you will have a solid understanding of the brain's critical role and why it is so important to train your brain once and for all.

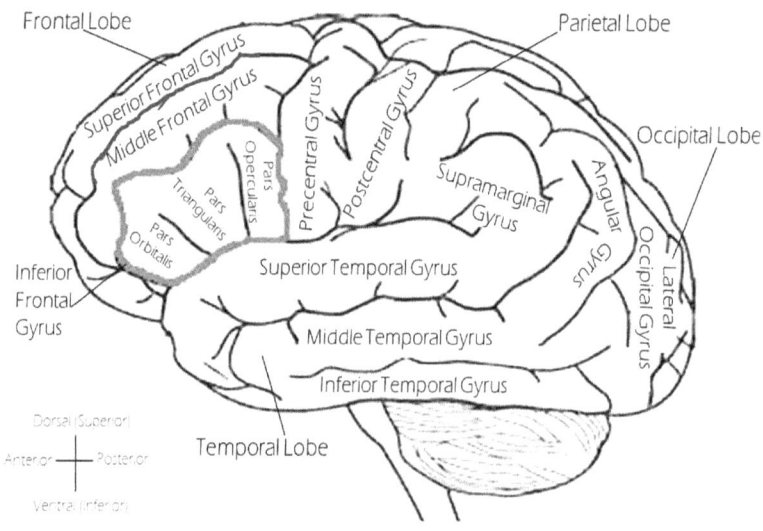

The Nervous System

Ultimately, the brain and all of the parts that are connected to it are known as the nervous system.
The nervous system can further be divided down into two forms: The central nervous system and the peripheral nervous system. Each nervous system has its own purpose. Ultimately, both nervous systems are comprised primarily of neurons
—the nerve cells within your body that allow for the exchanging of messages from neuron to neuron.

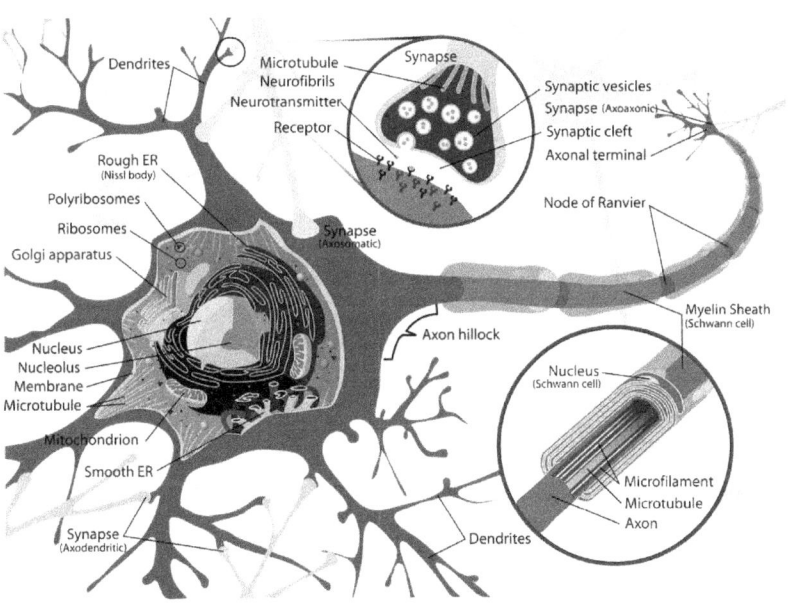

Your central nervous system is your brain and your spinal cord. This is where most of the heavy lifting is done
—your brain is responsible for thoughts and interpretations of the environment around you, while also being responsible for your actions.

Your spinal cord is what allows your brain to communicate with the rest of your body.

Your peripheral nervous system then is everything else. It is the rest of the nerves throughout your body, all of which eventually travel back to your brain.

These nerves are afferent when they carry down stimuli from the body to the brain for interpretation and processing. Efferent nerves, then, travel away from the central nervous system in order to trigger movement and sensation.

Neurons spread throughout the entire body.

They allow you to perceive the world around you, receiving input from the world, and then sending that input to the brain.

In the brain, the input is then translated and processed —your brain figures out how to respond to the stimulus that has been perceived by your body.

Your brain then sends out a command that tells your body how to handle it. For example, imagine that you have just touched a pan on the burner in your kitchen.

The nerves in your fingers register the sensation of intense heat, that understanding of pain is shot from the nerves in your fingers all the way up your arm, to your spine, and then to your brain.

Your brain then translates those impulses, decides to register it as pain, and sends the message back down to your fingertips —"PAIN! HOT! MOVE YOUR HAND!"

Then, you feel the pain, the pain triggers your response to pull away, and you do.

Now, imagine that message for everything:

you saw a blue bird fly by? That is sent to your brain for processing. The feeling of a cold breeze?

Your brain registers that as well.

Everything that you feel is going to be processed and registered by your brain.

The Brain's Central Role

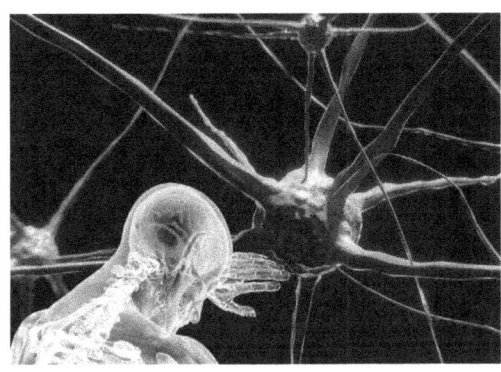

Within the central nervous system comes the brain. The brain is responsible for it all, as has been established. It controls and coordinates; it allows you to read, think, interact, and feel. It allows you to remember what happened yesterday and allows you to have certain feelings in response to what has happened. It makes you sad when you lose something, or angry when you are threatened.

Your brain is, effectively, everything you are.

The brain is incredibly specialized:

there is a specific area for every function you have in your brain.

Some parts are responsible for your speech

—one part for listening and understanding, and another for producing speech.

Other parts regulate your ability to breathe without even being conscious, while others still keep your heart beating.

Ultimately, your brain becomes the single most important part of your body.

The Left vs. the Right

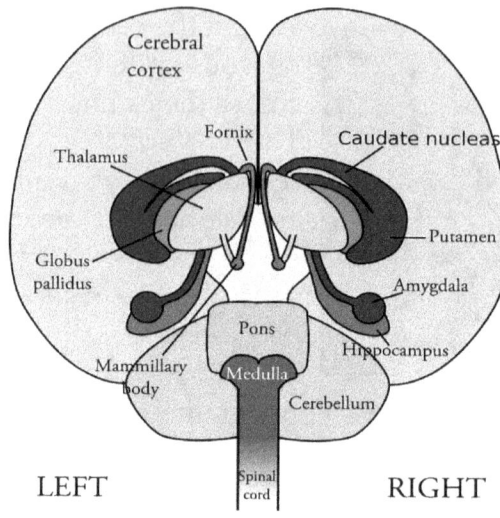

The brain's function is commonly divided into left and right brain functions.

The idea is that most people will favor one side of their brain over others:

— some people prefer to use their right side, and others prefer to use their left.

Understanding the difference can allow for some great insight into people, as well as how to understand how your own brain works.

When you can identify whether you are left or right brained, you will be able to better work with your own natural tendencies. Just as you would not hinder yourself if you were left-handed by making yourself use your right hand constantly, you should work with your own natural strengths and tendencies.

This theory asserts that people are going to be either more analytical or more creative.

The left brain is associated with methodical, analytical thinking that is designed to function on numbers, logic, and linear thinking, whereas the right brain is associated with the use of intuition and creativity.

This means that if you tend to think about and interact with the world through intuition, arts, and other imaginative, creative means that are not concrete logical numbers to back up your position, you are likely right-brained.

If you prefer to think in logical methods, following math and facts, you are likely left-brained.

Left Brain	Right Brain
• Logic • Sequences • Math • Linear thought processes • Factual thinking • Thinking in words	• Using imagination • Thinking holistically • Intuitive • Artistic • Rhythmic • Focusing on noverbal cues • Visualizing • Daydreaming

While you will always be using both sides of your brain all the time, thanks to a bundle of nerves called the corpus callosum. You may find that you do prefer one side over the other in terms of being able to solve problems.

Keep in mind that it is important to have both sides of your brain strengthened.

You should always make sure you exercise both your left and right brain processes in order to help yourself maintain and achieve maximum brain training.

Emotions and the Brain

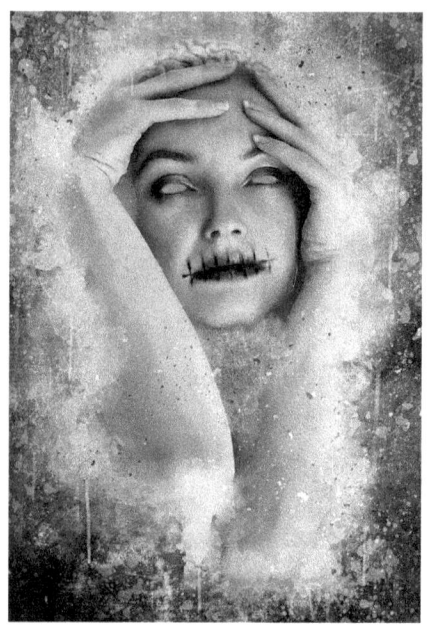

Of course, if your brain is responsible for everything that is you, that includes the creation of emotions. Your emotions serve very important roles in keeping you motivated, but they are also quite dangerous. They are great for getting you to move when you need to, allowing your brain to directly communicate quickly with your body in order to ensure that you are safe and able to live another day, but it usually comes at a cost.

People who are emotional rarely are able to make rational decisions.

While emotions have their place, they come at that cost. Consider acting in fear, for example. Your brain is telling your body right at that moment that it should flee from something that is threatening it: it is making the point that there is something dangerous and potentially fatal around you, and you must avoid it. When you are focusing on running away, you are not going to be thinking particularly clearly. Blood and functioning are diverted from your brain, where all of that rational thinking occurs, and instead is going to the keeping the heart pumping quicker, the lungs processing more oxygen, and the limbs to keep running.

Of course, that means that you are not able to think as much.
Your emotions become a distraction for you, and if you allow those emotions to take control of your body, you are beginning a battle between your body and mind and your emotions will almost always win unless you know how best to keep them wrangled.

Let's take a look at the seven universal emotions and their purposes for a moment.
These are known as universal because they have been identified in nearly every culture around the world, and people can universally recognize these emotions in others as well.
No matter whether you have grown up entirely isolated from other human beings or if you were surrounded by people, you will have these particular emotions and create the same sort of reaction to them.

These emotions are happiness, sadness, anger, fear, disgust, surprise, and contempt.

- **Happiness:**

    This emotion is what you feel when your needs are all met. It usually signifies to you that you have done something well and should keep doing that one particular thing because it is working well. For example, you may feel happy after eating good food, encouraging you to go and eat that food again in the future. It also allows you to relax and rest because you are not afraid or worried about meeting any needs.

- **Sadness:**

This emotion usually cues to you that you have done something that has caused hurt or pain. You may have lost something or someone, such as a family member, or you have done something that cost you dearly. When you feel sad, you are effectively feeling something negative to teach yourself not to do that one thing again. If you lost someone close to you, you might then decide to avoid that situation again, for example. It is the ultimate learning by negative feelings and consequences.

- **Anger:**

This emotion is directly related to feeling threatened. It is usually an offshoot of feeling fear and is your fight response kicking in. Most often, it conveys a need for space and boundaries, and if you cannot get it, you may find that you are far more likely to respond aggressively in order to get that space. You know that you need it to protect yourself.

- **Fear:**

This is the other emotion you are going to feel if you are threatened. However, fear has the potential to become anger if it is a situation in which the brain believes it can fight or fend off the threat. When the fight instinct is not triggered, however, the individual is likely to remain fearful, actively attempting to avoid the threat by running away.

When you are afraid, what you are looking for is protection or space away from whatever it is that is scaring or threatening you at that particular moment.

- **Disgust:**

This is the emotion you feel when you see something that is repulsive. Commonly considered with regard to seeing something rotting away, such as rancid meat or a rodent carrying disease, you feel disgust to spur yourself to avoid that particular stimulus. The smell of rotting meat, for example, is going to trigger that feeling of disgust, leading you to back away and avoid the meat, which would most likely make you sick if you were to consume it. Of course, you can also be disgusted at people and their actions as well, triggering a similar reaction and response. When something disgusts you, you will actively attempt to make space between yourself and that other object solely because it is repulsive to you.

- **Contempt:**

Contempt is a tricky feeling to define—it is somewhere between anger and disgust. When you feel contempt, you feel utter hatred and disdain toward whatever it is that is triggering those contemptuous feelings in the first place. Perhaps that contempt is felt toward someone who has repeatedly wronged you, such as an ex-partner who has cheated on you repeatedly.

- **Surprise:**

    When you feel like you are surprised, your mind is directly telling your body that something is not lining up quite right. Something that you have perceived violates the acceptable limits or expectations that you have. Think of how you would feel if, instead of falling, a ball floated up toward the ceiling when it rolled off of a table — you would be surprised because your expectation was not met. Likewise, when something around you, such as a spider being somewhere that you do not expect, shows up, you are going to be surprised. Surprise usually quickly transitions into one of the other emotions — you may feel surprise and then happiness at a surprise party, for example, or surprise and anger when someone cuts you off on the freeway, almost causing an accident.

With these emotions in mind, you should always be mindful of them causing problems for you in the future.
It is easy to get caught up in those emotions as they occur, triggering you to end up acting emotionally rather than rationally.
Keep in mind that if you do find that you tend to act emotionally instead of rationally, there are ways to work around this, and that is exactly what brain training will seek to do.

Stress and the Brain

Emotions are not the only drains of rational thought and 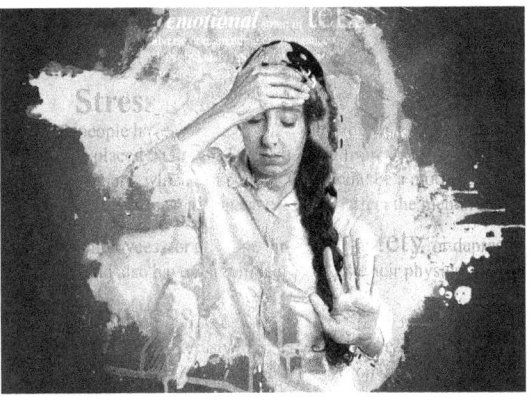 thinking abilities. Stress is another major destroyer of one's ability to think clearly. Stress is oftentimes accepted as an unfortunate part of life today—you may be stressed because you have work deadlines, or stressed because money is not stretching quite as far as it used to.

No matter the cause for stress, however, one thing is for sure: stress, especially when it becomes excessive, is detrimental.

Stress is defined as a response by the brain to any sort of demand, meaning that on its own, stress is not always negative or problematic: it is simply a response to something.

You will go through stress basically every time that you do anything. However, the intensity of that stress changes. In particular, we will be focusing on stress that actually becomes detrimental to brain function.

In particular, the top two stressors for adults are money and work.

Particularly in today's economic situation, people are always worrying about money. Life is getting expensive quickly: what used to cost a dollar may now cost two or three, and people are feeling that strain. The cost of living continues to skyrocket while people themselves do not see their own wages go up to accommodate. The cost of living continues to bypass their wages, and they feel stressed as a result of the inability to meet all of the demands.

When your body is stressed, a chain reaction occurs in the brain.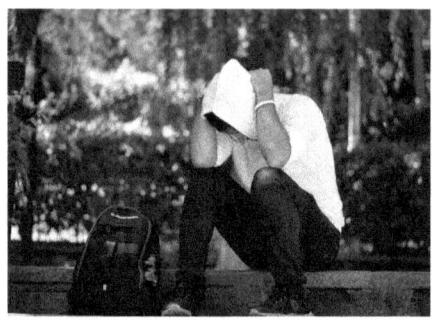
The amygdala, a part of the brain responsible for emotions, tells the hypothalamus that there is something stressful happening.
The hypothalamus then projects that message to the rest of the body, and before you know it, the fight or flight response has been triggered.
Your body feels like it is threatened, and while there may not be a saber-tooth tiger staring down at you from atop a rock, you still react with that same fear response. You still feel that same surge of adrenaline that increases your heart rate.
After that, adrenaline comes the cortisol—the hormone that is commonly attributed to stress.

Over time, if you never get a reprieve from all of that stress, you will find that there are serious long-term implications for your brain.
Cortisol, which is usually cleared out after the stressor has gone, is left to instead build up within the body. As it builds up, you see all sorts of other problems. The body is constantly building up cortisol, more than it needs, and the brain begins to see all sorts of negative results.

Stress has been found to reduce the size of the brain, shrinking the prefrontal cortex. This is the part of your brain that is necessary if you want to make good memories and learn. If your prefrontal cortex is directly impacted, you are going to find that you struggle in other areas as well. You will struggle to learn effectively, which means you can say goodbye to the possibility of ever actually being able to remember that shopping list or those chores that needed to get done.

Effectively, since stress triggers that reaction of fear and fight or flight within people, it is directly detrimental to the ability to rationalize. You will find those areas to be problematic, meaning that your own stress levels need to be regulated for your own sake.

The Importance of Sleep

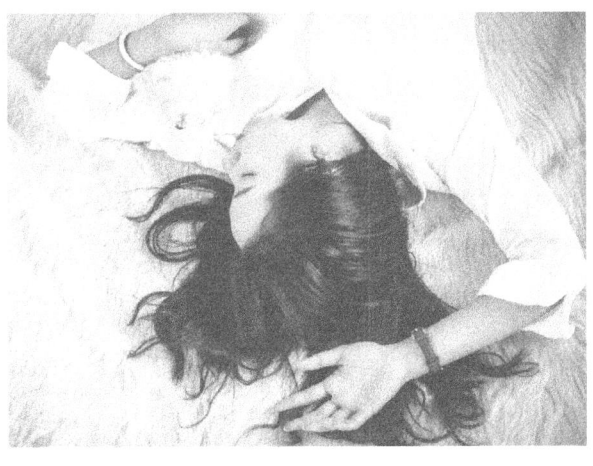

One last negative factor when you want your brain working optimally is looking at sleep. Not only do you need to be getting the right amount of sleep, but the sleep you are getting must also be the right kind of sleep as well.

Your body needs between 7 and 9 hours of sleep a night in order to get the right sort of balance of sleep for itself to optimize itself.

When you sleep, your body is repairing itself.

It allows energy to be restored to cells and allows waste byproducts from the brain to be cleared out as well.

This then also allows the brain to learn better. Sleep is also critical in regulating hormones that are responsible for your mood, your appetite, and even your sex drive.

Sleep occurs in two forms—you have slow-wave sleep, which is deep sleep, and rapid eye movement sleep, also known as dreaming sleep.

When you sleep, you are most often in short-wave sleep—the kind that keeps you in deep sleep. During this stage, your muscles are relaxed, and your breathing is deep and slow. This is believed to be the restful kind of sleep.

In rapid eye movement sleep, however, the opposite happens. Your body becomes paralyzed so it cannot act out the dreams that you are having. Your heart rate and breathing respond to your dreams as well.

We do not yet know why people have this sort of sleep, but what is known is that it is a vital part of your sleep cycle.

When you do not get this proper amount of sleep, you are going to feel bogged down and foggy. This is because your brain is tired—it did not get that rest; it needed to allow it to function at optimal performance.

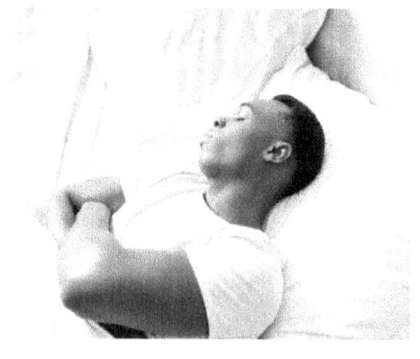

Your neurons are not going to function properly if they cannot rest when they need to, causing lapses in memory. As you get tired, your neurons begin to slow down and fire weaker than they usually do.

You will run into other issues as well—if you become sleep deprived enough, your brain will rest itself, with certain parts of the brain beginning to doze off while others are running.
This can lead to a lapse in memory or thought as parts of your brain shut down.

Of course, this has some pretty serious implications beyond just being able to remember lists—when you need a rapid reaction time, such as when driving, if you are sleep deprived, you will not have that.

If you are driving and a deer darts in front of you, your sleep deprived brain will take far longer to process it.
You are more likely to hit the deer than avoid it simply because your brain is not firing as rapidly as it normally would.
In fact, not sleeping enough can be compared to drinking alcohol—it causes the same sort of slowdown of the brain that can be incredibly problematic.

Chapter 2: Concentration

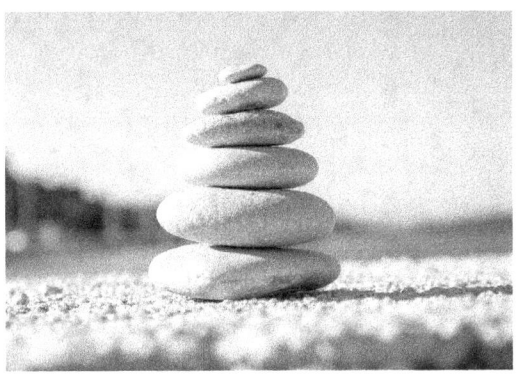

Have you ever watched an infant play with one of those shape sorters? The kind that has the shaped holes carved into the top with shaped blocks that only fit in the proper holes—these are commonplace in daycare rooms and nurseries everywhere.

Infants who are just beginning to figure out the world will play with this toy for far longer than you may think—they are concentrating.

Concentration is a critical skill for people to learn, and yet, people struggle with it around the world.

In a world designed around social media, constant distractions, and demand for multitasking, it becomes difficult to expect other people to actually be able to concentrate.

Within this chapter, we will take a look at what constitutes concentration, how to use it, why it matters, and how to improve it. It is a critical skill that everyone should have, and despite that, it is no longer the common presence that it used to be.

What is Concentration?

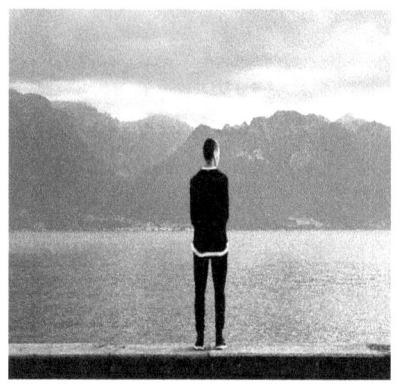

At its simplest, concentration is your ability to direct your attention where you want it, and keep it there as long as you want.

Effectively, it is your ability to control your thinking and attention exactly as you wish to do so. Even with distractions present, you are able to concentrate and focus, excluding those other thoughts and distractions from your conscious perception.

Concentration is rare these days because it involves the complete engrossment in just one task at a time, ignoring everything else.

Think of that infant that is purposefully trying to push that block through the correct hole—nothing else is catching the child's attention.

They do not care that there is a ball next to them, or that the other two children in the room are chasing each other, or even that their mother is nearby—the infant simply focuses on that one shape and figuring out how it fits.

Concentration, then, requires a kind of focus that is nearly impossible to achieve when you are readily available at all times around you.

If you are at work, for example, and keep your cell phone next to your computer so you can see the little LED notification blinking at you when you get a new email or message, you are not going to be able to focus on your work—you are going to be distracted.

The Importance of Concentration

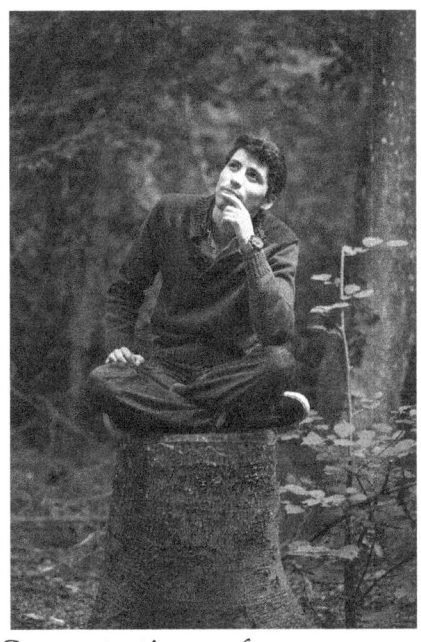

Concentration becomes important, then, because it allows for productivity.

When you can concentrate, you are not distracted by every pretty butterfly that passes your window, or by every little sound that you hear around you.

When you can concentrate, you can keep your attention where it needs to be, and that is something that people struggle with.

Concentrating, of course, means that you will not be reaching for your cell phone or checking your social media in the middle of your work day—you will instead be focused on whatever task you must complete.

When you concentrate, your mind becomes more powerful—it is focused and attentive, and that makes it productive and powerful. Your thoughts are regulated, allowing you to give each and every task the appropriate attention, and that gives you willpower.

When you are unwilling to be distracted by your lack of concentration, you are more likely to find that you do not have to force yourself back to attention. You will be able to influence yourself to become the person that you wish to be simply by being able to control yourself.

For example, imagine that you want to be able to achieve a new goal. Perhaps you want to learn to speak Japanese. When you want to learn something new, you need to be able to focus on it appropriately.
Some tasks may not need much attention—learning to spell a word in your native language, for example, may be quite easy, and after a time or two, you will find that it is no problem at all.
However, concentrating long enough to learn a language requires infinitely more attention simply due to the complexity.
When you are able to concentrate at will, however, you will be able to give that new language the attention it needs.

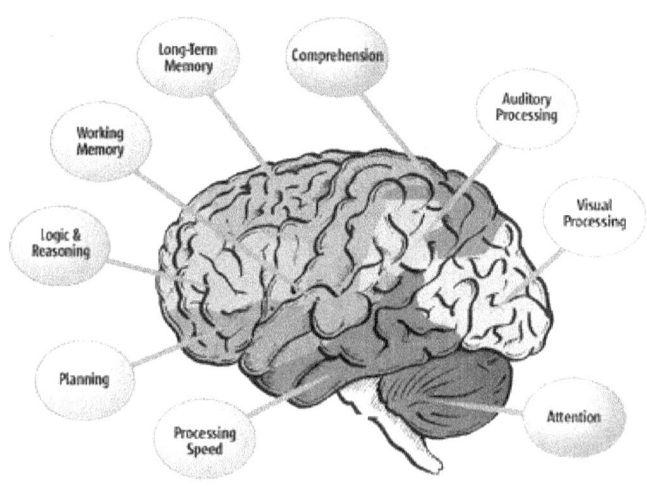

Improving Concentration

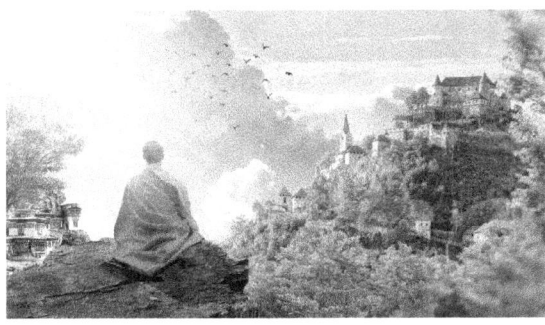

When you want to improve your concentration and develop that sort of willpower and attention where it needs to be, you need to strengthen your mind.

You need to develop that willpower so you can use it at will.

You need to have the strength to tell yourself to stay on task and not to get distracted by that new episode of your favorite television show, or that picture online of your best friend on vacation.

You need to be able to remind yourself what you are doing and why you are doing it, so you are not distracted.

Of course, this requires practice and focus of its own—it is not easily attained without the appropriate effort. Effectively, then, the way that you improve your own concentration is through repeated practice of being concentrated on something.

At first, you may find that you can only concentrate for short periods of time, but after a while, a few minutes will be easy. Soon, you will find that you can concentrate longer and longer. The trick, however, is repetition.

Think about how your workouts for your body are always repetitive—you do this because it is effective, and it works in concentration as well.

Concentration, Learning, and Forgetting

Think of your ability to learn as painting a picture. If you rush through the process, the paint will not dry appropriately.

In areas of the painting that have layers of colors, you will find that the colors mix and muddy instead of sitting nicely atop each other.

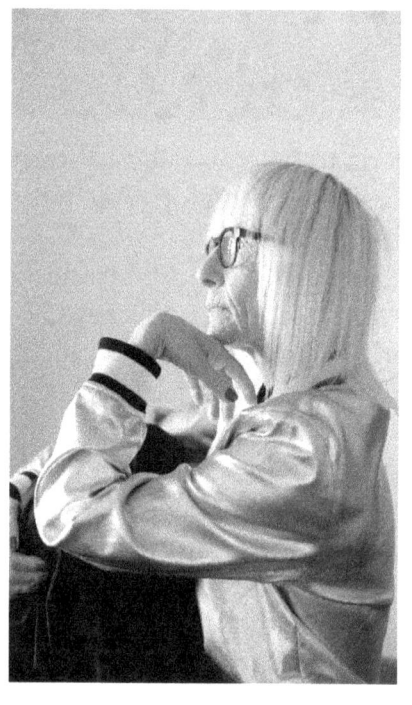

What could have been a nice, bright moon if it had been painted atop a dark background that had the proper amount of time to dry instead becomes a greyish blob on your sky because you never let the paint dry.

It may even begin to run together as the concentrations of paint build up.

If you let the colors dry, however, between layers, you will find that your painting is much more cohesive. You do not have colors bleeding together and instead get that nice, defined, clean picture that you were going for.

When you space out your learning, you are doing the same thing as spacing out the layers—you are letting those first neural networks set and begin to develop before attempting to reinforce them.

Being able to concentrate, then, is the ability to make sure that you are giving the appropriate amount of time to each and every layer of paint that you build up to create a solid masterpiece.

Similar to learning, however, comes forgetting.
When you are talking about memory, there are two factors to keep in mind—storage strength and retrieval strength.

Your storage strength is the information that has been recorded by the brain. It is how well you know the item, so to speak, and is what is strengthened with repetition and use. This is fixed from learning and only increases over time—it never decreases.

Your retrieval strength, on the other hand, is the ability to access that memory or thought. This does not last—it fades if you do not use something. If you forget something, it is not that the thought and information was lost forever or erased—instead, it is like losing the thought. Instead of having that beautiful, immaculate painting that you made through concentration destroyed in a fire, it is more like you put that painting in storage somewhere and then promptly forgot where it is.

This is why repetition is key—when you repeat something, you are not only strengthening the storage, but also increasing the retrieval strength. Doing so allows the brain to continue to remember that information without losing it.

The Repetition Method

To emphasize the effectiveness of repetition, let's look at a method for learning and concentration that makes use of that repetition.

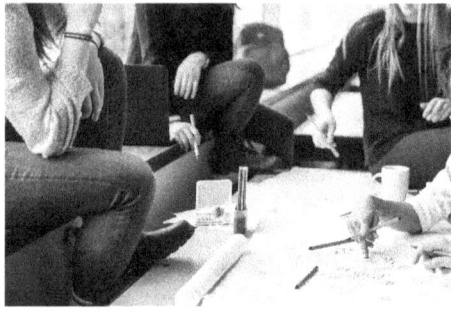

Here, we are considering a method of studying or work that will space out the time that you are focusing. First of all, repetition over time has the added benefit of being, well, repetitive.

You are going to learn things better the more times you practice them. Just as your body develops the appropriate muscles in response to repetitive workouts, you will find that your brain will develop the appropriate neural connections through repetition as well.

However, there is another benefit to this repetitive method of learning and training the brain—when you are using analysis, or other higher level brain functions, spacing it out allows for those neural connections, which will be more complex than, for example, learning the spelling of a new word, time to be reinforced over time.

Let's stop and look at exactly how you can maximize out this learning through repetition.
There is actually an optimal interval spacing that you can use to really learn the information. Through research and repetition practice and experiments, the optimal intervals have actually been found.

Of course, the optimal intervals for repetitive studying do depend and vary somewhat based on the time that you have available—for example, if you have a year to study for a test, you have many more opportunities for timed intervals. However, let's look at the simplified version. To maximize learning potential, you want to use the following intervals:

- Study
- Wait one day
- Study
- Wait 7 days
- Study
- Wait 16 days
- Study
- Wait 35 days
- Study

This spacing allows you to repeatedly reinforce the learning of the material over time.

Of course, you will still need to revisit this material sometimes if you really hope to learn it and make sure it sticks for a lifetime, as if you do not use it, you lose it, but if you follow patterns like this, repeating your studying of the object or item, you will find that you are able to better remember the material long-term.

Chapter 3: Association

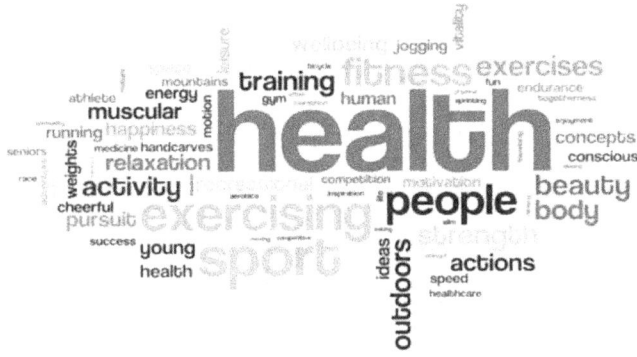

Did you ever hear any silly tricks to learn random facts in school?

Maybe you heard the mnemonic;

Every Good Boy Deserves Fudge in music class when you were learning to read sheet music as a way to remember the order of the lines on the bar.

Perhaps you took that Japanese class in high school, and your teacher emphasized that you could remember how to say "You're welcome," by remembering the phrase, "Don't touch my moustache," to trigger the memory of the phrase, "Douitashimashite," which is quite the mouthful for someone just learning the language.

Maybe you heard that Italy is the boot of Europe in order to remember where it is on a map.

Maybe the only thing you remember about cellular biology is that the mitochondria are the powerhouse of the cell, simply because of the imagery it brought with it back in 10th grade biology. All of these are examples of ways that you can boost your memory by association.

This trick is commonly used in schools and classes.

When something is tricky to learn, teachers everywhere love to make use of associations that can make that learning just a bit easier. For example, you may remember the most useless knowledge now simply because it was put to something that was memorable in school.

This makes it powerful—you create something so memorable that it is hard to forget it.

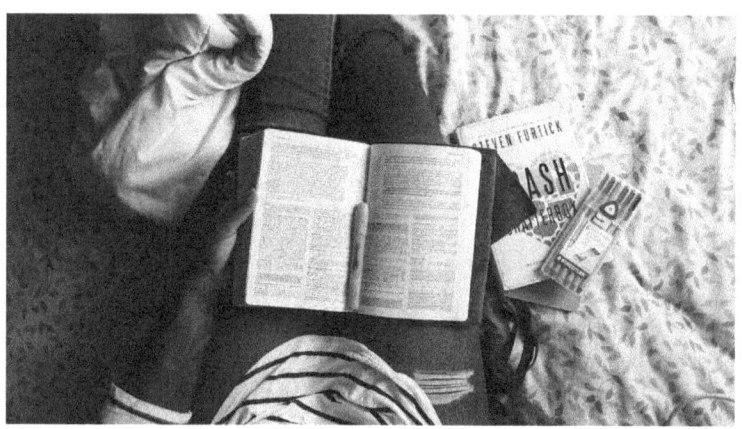

Within this chapter, we will be looking at association in depth. You will learn how learning through association is so powerful, and why it is commonly used.

You will also be introduced to a few methods of using association, as well as how to do so.

When you finish reading this chapter, you should find that you are far more capable of creating these associations to better boost your own ability to remember and recall information that is important for you to learn.

If you need to study for a test, this method will work for you. If you are trying to learn a name or a place, this will work for you. Even learning phone numbers or addresses can be boosted through this method.

Learning by Association

When you create an association for yourself, you are effectively allowing yourself to have an easier way to recall something.

You are effectively creating a new cue for yourself to trigger that particular bit of information that you need.

If you are stuck in your Japanese class and cannot remember how to say you're welcome when your teacher thanks you, you may freeze up.

You feel like the word is on the tip of your tongue, and yet you cannot recall it.

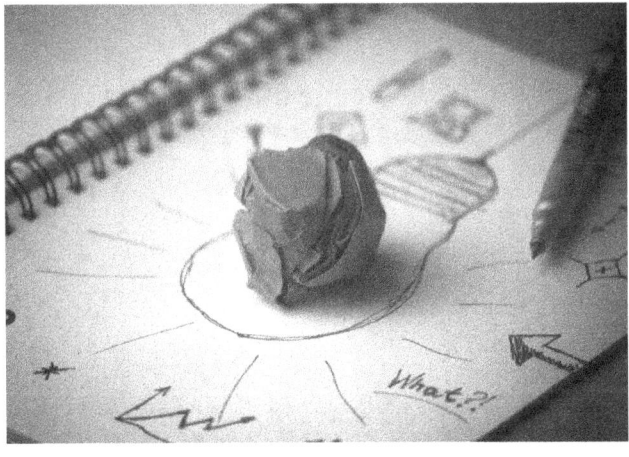

However, when you have some sort of association that you have paired to it, you can then rely on that association instead. Rather than awkwardly responding in English, you could, for example, tell yourself, "don't touch my mustache," in order to remind yourself. Then, you are able to trigger that memory. Suddenly, you remember exactly how to utter the phrase in Japanese; you do so, avoid embarrassment, and everyone in class cheers.

Okay, maybe they don't cheer, but you will be mentally cheering yourself on for creating the mnemonic in the first place.

Eventually, you will no longer need that imagery for your memory. You may not need to tell yourself to lay off the mustache in order to say you're welcome in Japanese, but you are far more likely to remember how to say it in 10 years of not using the language at all than you would be to ask some other, much more specific question or phrase, all because that mnemonic is still there for you.

Simply being able to recall that mnemonic allows you to have an extra sort of string to that particular piece of information in your mind — it basically bookmarks it as having another method that can be used to recall it. Instead of having to rely on some other method, such as using a search engine or dictionary, you can simply remind yourself of your silly image that you used.

How Association Works

Association works primarily because you are able to follow three steps to create a mental link. In forming that mental link and making sure that you have a method through which you can recall that information at will, you are making the recall power of that particular bit of information far higher.

Taking advantage of association skills is the perfect way to begin boosting your own abilities to register information quickly and effectively.

You will be more likely to recall the information simply because you have made it so memorable and different, and this means that this is one of the most effective, simplest methods that you can use.

When you use association, you are effectively forcing yourself to concentrate.

You are making yourself have to focus on that particular information enough to actively manipulate it into something else. After all, you cannot come up with the mnemonic, "My Very Educated Mother Just Showed Us Nine Planets" without knowing the planets. Of course, today, that is an outdated mnemonic, but if you went to elementary school before 2006, you likely remember that method of remembering the order of the planets. Nowadays, very educated mothers are serving nachos instead of showing nine planets with Pluto being demoted, but the method remains the same—you had to know the material to turn it into that mnemonic.

Using Association

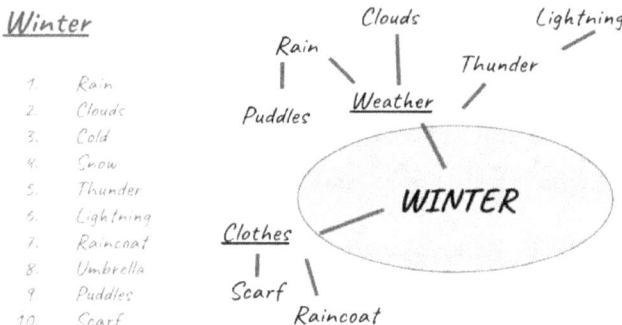

Winter
1. Rain
2. Clouds
3. Cold
4. Snow
5. Thunder
6. Lightning
7. Raincoat
8. Umbrella
9. Puddles
10. Scarf

When you decide to use association, you are going to be using three specific steps.
When you use these steps, you can come up with your own basic mental links that will help you learn the information that you need to learn.

First, let's consider what association is—it is creating a connection between two things.
Most of the time, those connections are made through visualization or through hearing. You may be able to visualize that Italy is shaped like a boot, allowing you to more or less draw the shape of Italy on demand, but would you also be able to draw a picture of China on demand? What about Nepal or France? You remember Italy simply because you associate it with a boot—something you can visualize.

Other times, you use the sound of something.
You know that douitashimashite sounds like don't touch my mustache, and don't touch my mustache is easier to remember in English when you are presumably already fluent.

These are both examples of making use of the first step of association: Using a substitute to cue or break down the concept. You are substituting the image of Italy for a boot, and the sound of the Japanese word for "Don't touch my mustache."

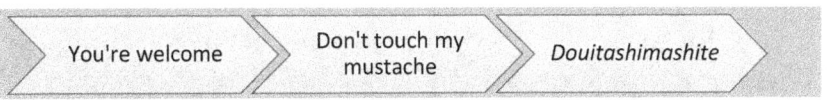

Next, after making that first association between the two, you must be able to link the image together.
You may force yourself to look at a map and think of Italy as a boot on the foot of the continent of Europe, or remind yourself several times as you go over your Japanese study material that you must remember to tell someone to leave your mustache alone.
As you visualize someone guarding their mustache as they say you're welcome in Japanese, you remember how to say it better and better.
Perhaps, you even stroke your own pretend mustache as you repeat the word to yourself, further emphasizing the likelihood of you remembering it later.

Finally, you will find that the associations are made. You are imagining that person protecting his mustache as he says you're welcome.
You imagine that boot on the foot of Europe. With that in mind, you eventually solidify the information.
Then, when you need to go to class, you can recall the information far easier.

Association Through Sounds

When you need to remember something tricky for class, perhaps the easiest way is to find something silly that relates to it.

If you, for example, need to remember what the capital of Washington State is, which is Olympia, for those who do not know, perhaps you break down the word, Olympia. Stop and consider the name of Washington. Instead of looking at the name and thinking of George Washington, look at the name of the state and think of the word, "Wash."

This brings the imagery of wetness, which Washington has plenty of, considering all of the rain that the Pacific Northwest gets.

Keeping the word wash in mind, you must then think of what happens to pie when it gets wet—it gets soggy, or limp.

In response, you say, "Oh, limp pie" in your displeasure or disgust.

This helps you remember, then, that the capital of rainy Washington is, in fact, Olympia.

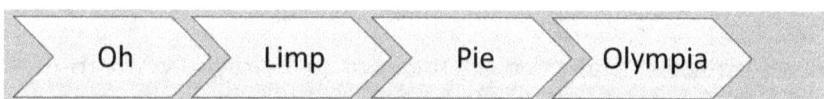

Association by Song

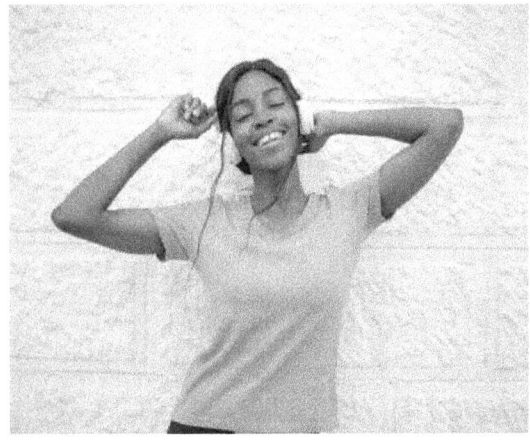

Another common method to help people learn information is to put it to a song of some sort.

A very common example of this seen in high school is through the use of the Quadratic Formula Song, which is the quadratic formula put to the tune of "Pop Goes the Weasel" in order to cue students to remember it.

The song is catchy enough to get stuck in their heads, and they never forget it. Other examples include the States song to remember the states, or the days of the week for preschoolers to help them learn them all.

When you want to do this, the best trick is to pick a melody that you know or is familiar with and then figure out how to put what you need to remember to the tune of that song.

Repeat the song to yourself a few times, and you may find that the information gets far easier over time.

The more you repeat it, the more likely you are to actually latch onto the memory and commit it for yourself, meaning that you will be far more likely to be able to access it later

Chapter 4: Connections

How often, when you are learning something, do you suddenly relate it to something else that you know how to do well?

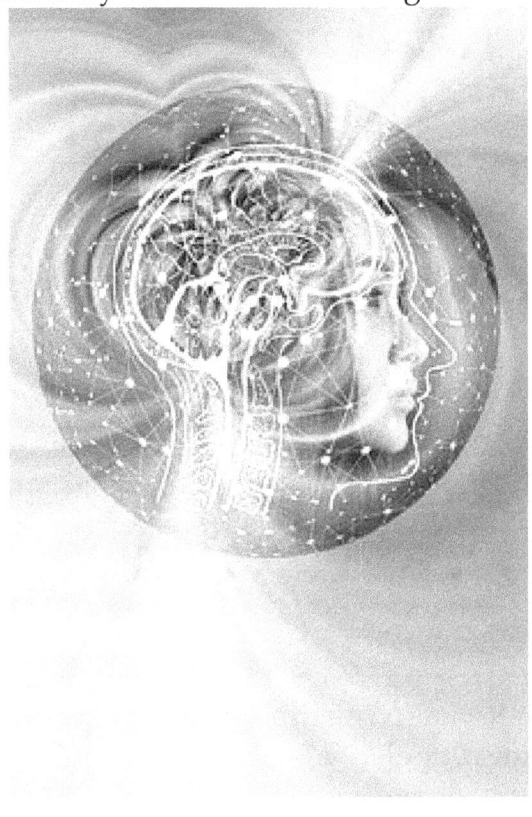

Perhaps you wanted to learn how to make cinnamon rolls, and you relate it to the process of making breadsticks— something you are intricately familiar with.

Maybe you were trying to learn how to say something in a foreign language and found that it actually shared a grammatical pattern with a language that you already know, or you chose to learn an instrument that was incredibly similar to one that you already learned before.

In all of these instances, you have some sort of background or prior knowledge that then makes the learning process that much simpler for you.

Instead of having to stress over how best to activate that information for yourself, you are able to connect it to

49

something else that you already know, making it so much more memorable.

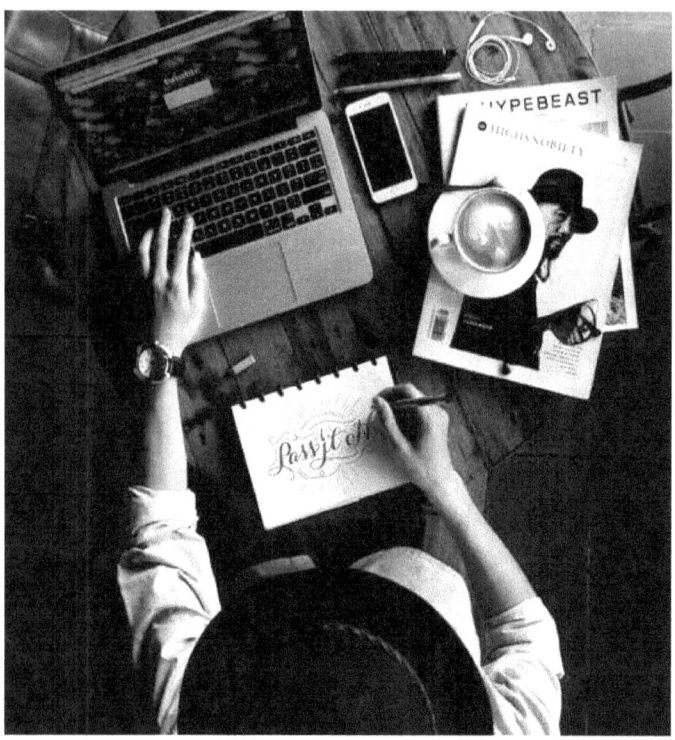

This is effectively making use of associations, but instead of associating the information with something new, you are relating it to something that you already remembered or knew from something else.

This is incredibly effective and is exactly why, especially in school, information is usually given in a specific order. After all, it is much easier to understand multiplication if you take it as addition repeated over and over again.

If you tried to learn multiplication without being able to make that connection to addition, you are more likely to struggle than someone who understands that process and acknowledges the similarities.

Making Connections

Making connections takes something away from being arbitrary knowledge and gives it some sort of root in your mind.
When you are activating connections between things, such as learning a new word through connecting it to one that you already know, relating the root word to it, you are able to make things more memorable for yourself.
You effectively allow it to be related information, which is a bit easier to recall than information that is otherwise floating on its own, unrelated to anything else that is being discussed at the moment.

Imagine, for example, that you are in a science class in college and just were introduced to the concept of "igneous" rocks. You do not know what they are, but when your professor mentions that they are rocks formed from magma and lava, you immediately relate it to the word "ignite," allowing for that connection in order to remind yourself that they are related to fire—or in this case, lava.

Of course, you can use this in other contexts as well.
If you are making lasagna for dinner and need to remember the seasoning that you are going to need to pick up, perhaps you remind yourself that it needs most of the seasoning that you usually use for your spaghetti sauce as well—making that connection means that you do not need to check the recipe for that lasagna a dozen times at the grocery store and you get all of the seasonings that you need simply because you were able to connect the recipe to one that you already used regularly

Boosting Focus with Connections

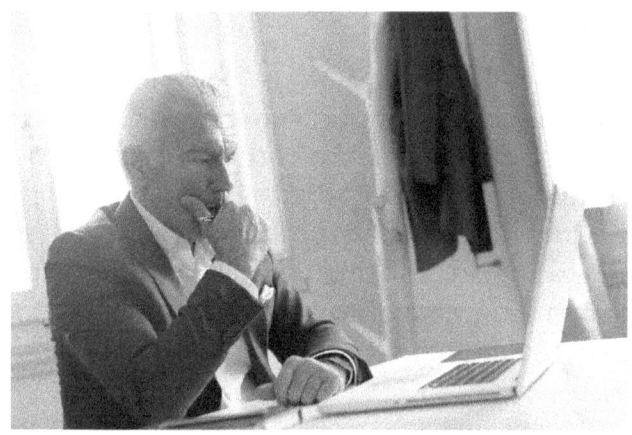

Of course, you can make connections to nearly anything, so long as it works for you. You can even make connections to memories to stimuli around you as well, allowing yourself to effectively trigger yourself to remember information with your environment.

You could, for example, study to music that you like in order to help you focus.

If you like the music that is playing, you are far more likely to focus strongly, regardless of whether the music has lyrics or not. All that matters is whether you like the music that you are playing.

You may also choose to create a specific association between a certain stimulus and that thought process.

For example, maybe you make your to-do list while chewing spearmint gum.

Then, when you chew spearmint gum, later on, you are more likely to recall the information simply because you are recreating the sensations within your body that were present when you were making that to-do list in the first place.

Making connections is quite powerful, so long as you are doing so intentionally.

You may relate information to yourself and your own life—perhaps remembering that someone else's birthday is on the same day as your own birthday, allowing you to create a sort of anchor point that helps you remember it.

You may use that musical connection to help you focus, playing the same soundtrack when you need to work to boost your productivity.

When your body hears that music, your brain will automatically trigger that sensation of being ready to be productive

Using Connections

Ultimately, making those connections usually comes in one of three forms—you relate the information to yourself, you relate the information to the world, or you relate the information to other information that you already know.

This means that you are making a connection between the new information and some sort of prior knowledge through firsthand, secondhand, or even third hand experience.

When you relate or connect information to yourself and what you have done or learned in life, it is usually quite memorable.

You may remember that birthday of your coworker because it is the birthday of your best friend or of your child.

You may remember that your best friend also hates peas because you hate peas, and you both joked about it at some point during an early conversation.

This is perhaps the easiest of the three to use — after all, what do you know better than yourself?

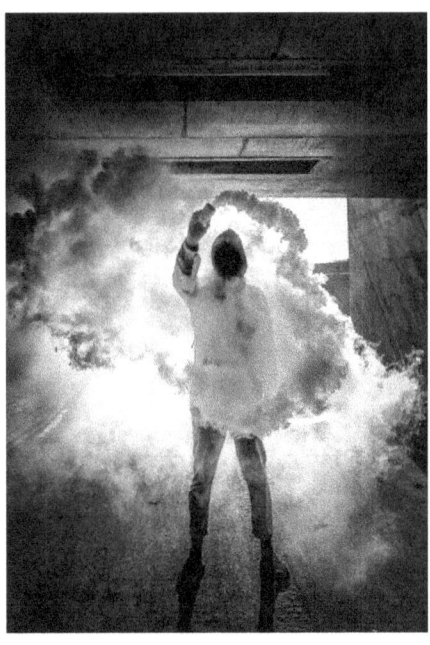

When you relate information to the world or your environment, you are creating a connection between something that has been experienced in order to remember it better.

By pairing up something new and unexpected with an older result or situation where something similar happened, you are able to better figure out how to deal with the problem or work through the situation.

For example, instead of panicking when you go to walk to your car and see a bear staring down the driveway at you, you stop and remember what you were taught to do when approached by a strange dog.

Instead of panicking, you are able to think clearly and logically and figure out what is best to do in that situation.

When you relate information to other background knowledge that you have on a situation, you make it more memorable simply because you know of another similar instance.

You may find that, for example, you stumble across a new word, and you are able to decipher it by relating it to other similar root words.

You can remember the ingredients to your recipe by relating them to a recipe that you are more familiar with.

Making Connections in Practice

When you need to connect a new piece of information to something more familiar to you, the best way to do so is most often through figuring out exactly how it does relate to something else that you know or are familiar with. Perhaps, instead of freezing up or trying to repeat it to yourself to remember, you try to come up with something that is relatable.

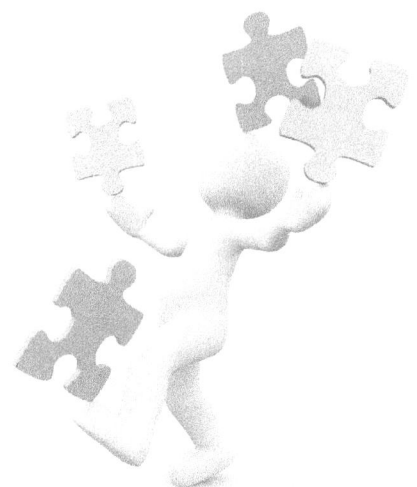

if you need to remember the date of your next appointment and do not have a calendar, for example, you would want to connect that data to something that is familiar. Perhaps you need to set your appointment for May 2 at 3:00pm. You know that you are not going to remember that if you simply leave it like that in your mind. However, what you will remember is pointing out that the appointment is the day after that birthday party that your child is going to. Suddenly, you can effectively anchor that appointment to something else on your schedule, making it a bit easier to remember without being able to write it down.

Now, instead of stressing out, you can tell yourself that the appointment is the day after your child's friend's birthday party at 3pm.

Of course, you can make connections to anything necessary.

All that is important is that you are anchoring that new information to something else to make it more memorable for yourself, allowing yourself to better remember it when you need it.

If you can do this, you will effectively boost the chances of you actively and accurately remembering that information as needed.

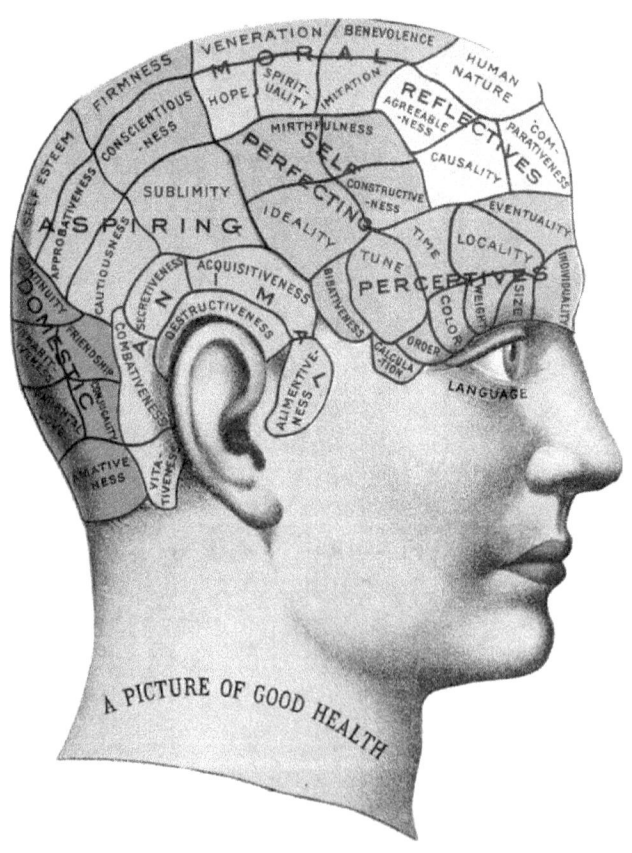

Chapter 5: Photographic Memory

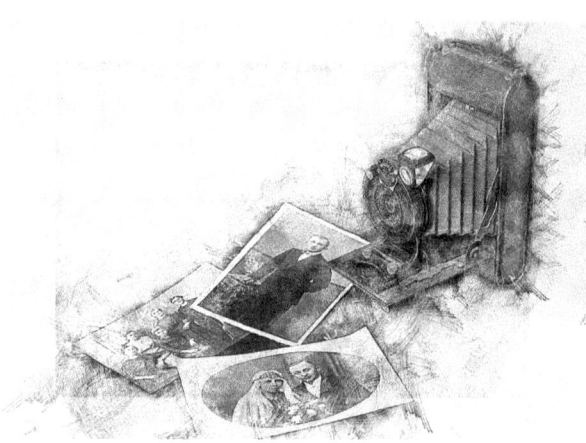

Imagine that your child has just come up to you and asked you where his shoes are. He needs them for soccer practice— which you are officially late for, and he has no idea where he left them. His room is a mess, your living room looks like a toddler tornado decimated any sense of organization, and you needed to leave 10 minutes ago.

Instead of stressing out, however, you can see that image of your child's shoes somehow in your mind's eye—you see them next to the discarded toy bat and fire truck in the living room and tell your child as such.

Sure enough, when he goes to look, the shoes are there, and he is in awe of your ability, declaring that you must be psychic or magic.

Are you? Not at all—however, you have a knack for visual memories. When you see something, even if you feel it is not particularly important, you seem to commit it to memory it somehow.

What is Photographic Memory?

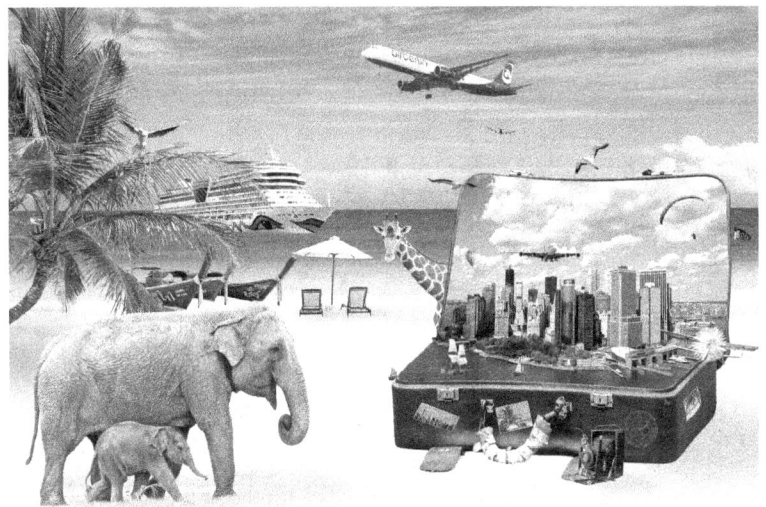

It is important to note that a truly photographic memory, the idea that you can simply create a mental snapshot of the world around you and have it clearly portrayed in your mind, does not exist.

No matter how good of a visual memory that you have, it will never be truly photographic. However, what we commonly refer to as photographic is also known as eidetic.

This is the ability to see an object in your mind after looking away from it. Some people have it to some degree, but it is rarely developed to its fullest potential. This form of memory is difficult to truly master.

While we all have an eidetic memory, it is usually not particularly honed—the image fades away after a few seconds.

However, for other people, the photograph or snapshot of that image is able to be recalled far longer. This is what is referred to as photographic—the image of that item is transferred to long-term memory instead of hanging out behind in short-term memory.

This memory works simply because when you see something, your brain has to do something with that image.

If it is not particularly memorable, such as the way that the road looked as you crossed the street somewhere on a perfectly ordinary day with nothing out of place, you are not going to be likely to keep the memory. It gets dumped. If it is somewhat memorable, such as if you saw an interesting car as you crossed the street, it may move to your short-term memory.

When it gets to short-term memory, your brain can either recall that memory, transfer it to long-term memory, or discard it.

Keep in mind that for most people, the image itself is not what is recorded.

You may remember the data, such as being able to recall that you saw the shoe by the bat, or that you saw 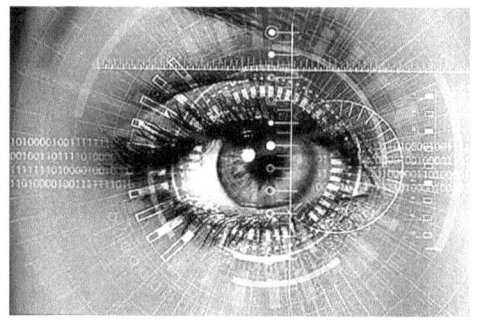 that car as you crossed the street, but you do not have that image painted in your mind the way that you saw it just moments before.

Developing a Photographic Memory

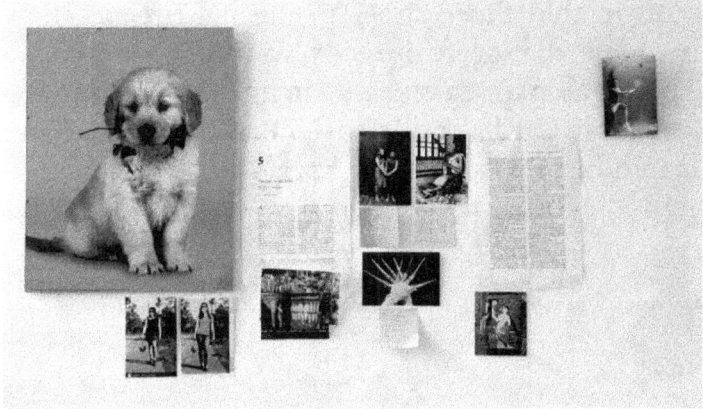

Despite the rarity, many people wish that they could develop this sort of memory.
Keep in mind, as a full disclaimer, that not everyone will be able to develop the photographic memory that they want.
Nevertheless, you can boost your memory in order to better take those pictures in your mind that you wish to create.

When you want to boost your photographic memory, you must first improve your memory. You want to train your brain, which, if you are reading this book, you are already well on your way to doing.
As you do so, you are able to keep your brain more limber and able to make those images that you wish to create.
You want to make sure that your mind is used to remembering strings of data, numbers, and words before you can ever hope to use it to remember photographs.

When you train your mind, one way to do so is to create associations through visualization, which will be discussed later within this book, or through actively associating what you see with other ways to remember. Perhaps you related those shoes to the bat because they were both items that were directly related to sports, so you were better able to register that image in your mind.

You can also use cards and card games to practice and train your mind.

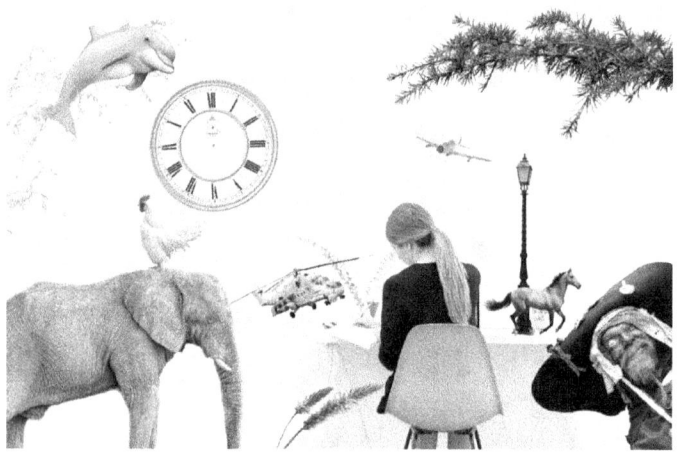

In doing so, making yourself remember where cards are or what they were, you are able to practice your own ability to memorize.

Perhaps you play memory with yourself with an entire deck of cards every day, keeping them in the same place at first until you have the placements memorized, and then you can change them again.

The whole purpose of doing so is simply to help you remember the information better and more accurately over time.

How Photographic Memory Boosts Focus

A photographic memory can greatly improve your ability to focus.

Usually, those who have a photographic memory in the first place claim that they are more confident, which can usually help them actively focus better and with less distractions.

If you are able to be confident in yourself, you are not likely to be distracted by worrying about whether you have done something the right way or worrying about embarrassing yourself.

Beyond that, however, you may also find that you are more able to focus in general simply because you have trained your brain to focus on the details in such great length. You may find that you can focus quicker on the details, painting that mental image far quicker than other people would be able to do so simply because you are practiced and well-versed in doing so.

You find that you can read quicker and more accurately than before as well simply because you have gotten so good at taking in the visual stimuli and processing it quickly.

This means that you will find that your own memory abilities go up dramatically, and that can only help your focus more in the future.

Because you are able to focus more on the world around you and on the information that has been provided in front of you, you will find that you are that much more prepared to focus in the future.

You strengthen that mental muscle and build that skill through rote practice, and this is just another way to flex those mental abilities.

The Military Method for Photographic Memory

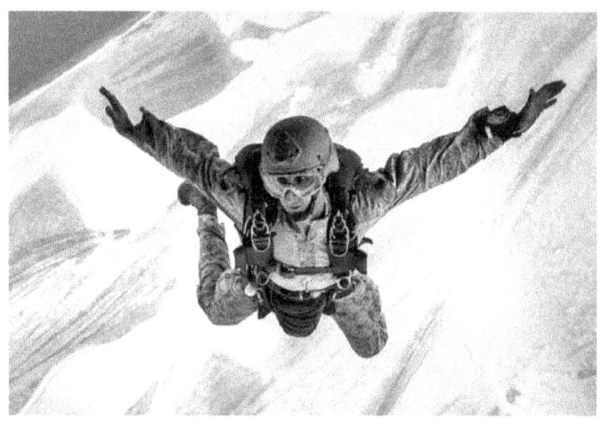

One method that people use to develop photographic memory is known as the military method. This is believed to be the method that militaries use to train operatives, though there has been no official confirmation on that fact.

However, whether it is used by the military or not, it is successful in improving the memory of people and getting one step closer to developing that coveted photographic memory.

Keep in mind that this method is time-consuming—in fact, it will take roughly a month to finish, and you must be able to commit to using it daily for that month in order to actually get that progress. If you do not practice daily, you are likely to set yourself back significantly. Despite the fact that it is daily, however, it only takes about 15 minutes every single day in order to get the process rolling and to see those results that you desire.

Start by setting yourself up in a dark room that is distraction-free.

Preferably, you should use a room without windows, or if you do not have that access, a room with blackout curtains in the evening hours when it is dark.
You may find that you can use a bathroom that has a ceiling light if you do not have any other options.

Take a book and a piece of paper. You want to cut a square into the paper that will frame a paragraph within the book.
The book here does not matter so much, so long as it is one that you are interested in reading daily for a month. Now, set the paper onto the book, framing just one paragraph. Make sure that it is a decent length for you, not just a paragraph with one or two sentences.

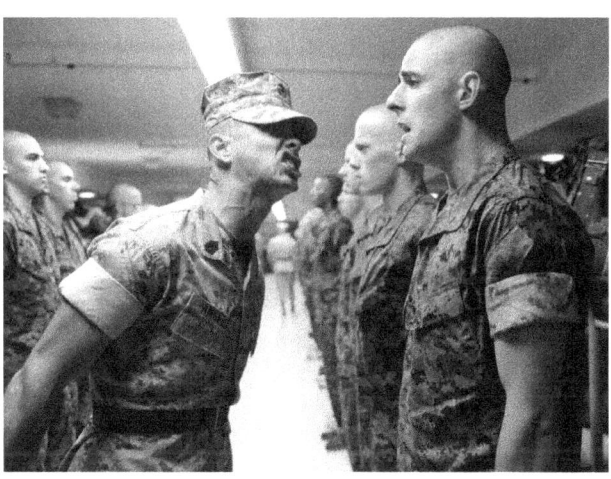

Now, figure out the right space in which the words of the paragraph are easily read at a glance. With the book in place and the paragraph framed, turn off the light and wait until you adjust to the lack of light. Then, you want to turn on the light quickly for a second as you look at the paragraph in front of you.
The light should only be on for about a second before you turn it off again. You then want to take that visual

impression in your mind and try to visualize it as long as you can.

As the image fades away, repeat the flickering of the light on and off again.

You will go through this process for about 15 minutes daily for a month until you can recall the order of the words in the paragraph.

You want to use the same paragraph every single day until you are able to recall it. Even if, at the end of the month, you cannot remember the whole paragraph, you should find that you have some of it memorized and that your own abilities to memorize and visualize are getting better.

Of course, you can use this method for longer than a month, too until you are satisfied with your own abilities to read the paper in front of you.

No matter how long you choose to do it, however, make sure you commit for at least 15 minutes a day for at least one whole month if you want to get the best results.

Chapter 6: Mind Maps

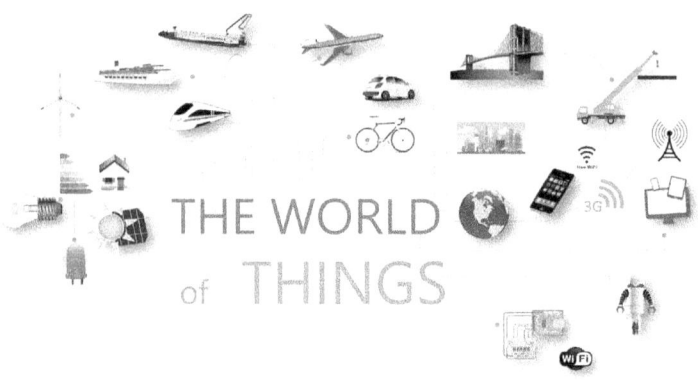

Have you ever felt like you had a fantastic idea in your mind, but you could not figure out how to get it organized enough to get it all out?

Maybe you like to write, and you have this great idea for your next novel, but you do not know how to make it actually make sense on paper.

After all, a stream of consciousness narration of everything that you were thinking would be incredibly unorganized and difficult to parse through in the future.

For times like these, when you need to figure out how best to address the organization of your information in your mind, mind maps can be critically important.

They can allow you to take notes of everything going on in your mind, allowing you to map it out once and for all, finally freeing your mind of the thoughts that may otherwise have been consuming you.

Discovering Mind Maps

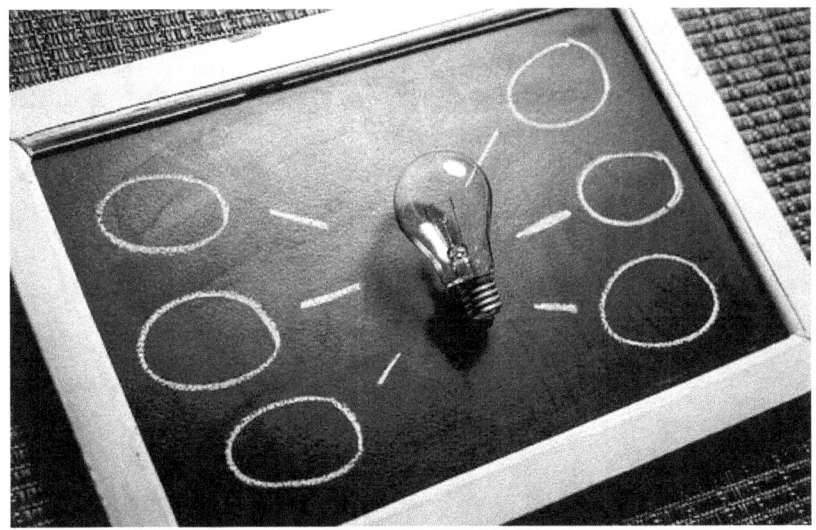

Mind maps share a few things in common — they are organized by nature thanks to their structure.

They start at a central idea and slowly branch out in several other directions. You can make them as colorful or monochromatic as you want.

They can be made up of data, words, pictures, or anything else that you have in your mind. They can also make space for all sorts of information all at once.

If you know that your mind tends to go a thousand different directions all at once, a mind map can be a great way to make sure that you are able to see how everything relates to each other.

Effectively, you can think of your mind map as a city.
At the center of the city is the main idea.
All roads in your city will be directed toward this central point. From there, you will have roads that branch off

from the city center, representing other, secondary thoughts.

These roads can continue to branch off, eventually giving yourself dozens or even more possible routes to get to the city's center, and you are able to see all of the information all lined out for yourself.

The greatest benefit of this sort of planning and organizing is that you can do things in any order you want. Because you will constantly be making new branches and offshoots of the thought, you will be able to begin at any thought that relates to that central thought and go back to it later.

Unlike with traditional notes, where you might run out of space, you will be able to simply branch off of it.

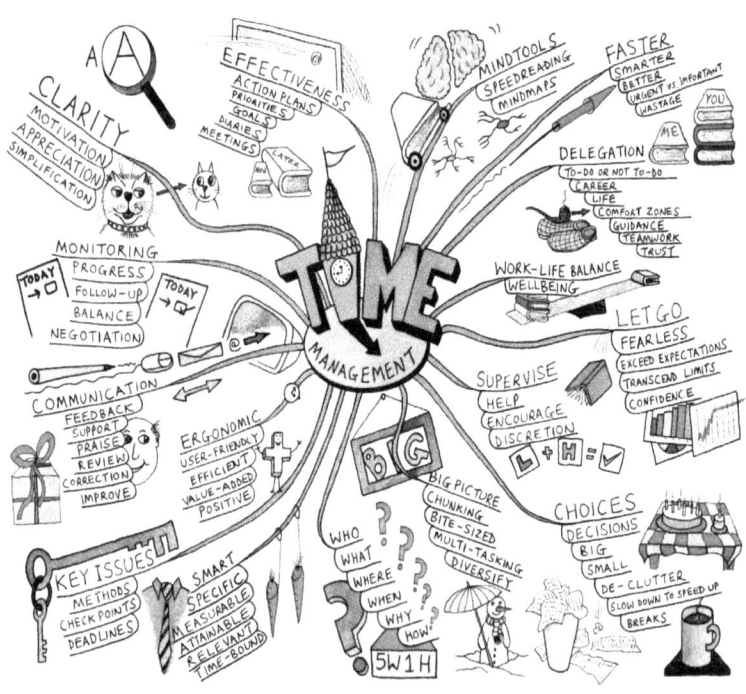

How Mind Maps Work

Mind maps work primarily because you are able to make them in any order with as many thoughts as you have, or do not have.

You can actively change and follow your thought processes as they happen, allowing yourself special insight into your mind.

Imagine that you are writing that novel mentioned earlier—you can see how everything plots around that main central theme that you have going on, and you are free to add to it as much as you want to without ever influencing the placement of anything else.

When mind maps are used, they allow people to follow their thoughts visually.

For those who may struggle to walk through everything in their minds, being able to see it all written out in front of them can actually be incredibly beneficial to them.

Ultimately, mind maps have five key components, but at the end of the day, what is more important is that you are making a structure that works best for you.

If you happen to be skilled in recognizing patterns or understanding how best to interact with your thoughts, then you may want to make it a point to change up how you want to do this. If you want to have thoughts that can diverge and come back together later, you can do that, too.

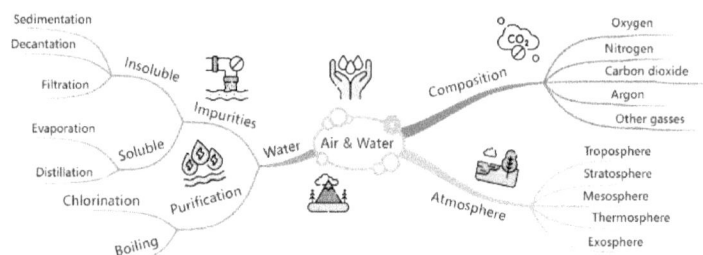

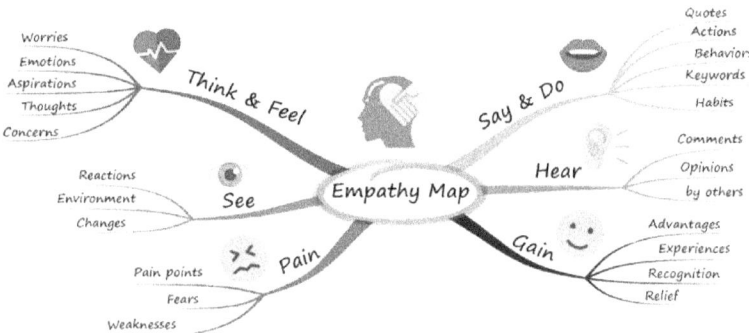

However, let's take a look at those five essential components.

- **The main idea is in the center (the tree):**

    Whatever the purpose of your mind map is must be at the center. This is your city center, or in this case, will be represented by your tree.

- **The main themes of the idea connect to the center (the branches):**

    Trees naturally have branches that shoot out from their main trunk. This is just how trees work, and your mind map will work the same way as well. Make sure that any related information is connected to the center.

- **The branches each make up their own key points:**

    Each branch that you include should be a major reference point for that center tree. They should all be directly related somehow and relevant enough to warrant their own key points.

- **Lesser important themes branch off of the branches (the twigs):**

    Sometimes, you have other themes that you must entertain, and this is where twigs come in. When your key points also have points to consider, they go onto branches.

- **The twigs must connect to the branches somehow:**

73

It is important to note that, when you are making your mind map, there must be some way that you can connect all twigs back to the main tree somehow. They may connect onto a branch, and if they do not connect to a branch, they may deserve their own branch. If the twig you are looking for a place to plant does not fit into either a branch or as a twig, it may not actually be relevant to your central idea.

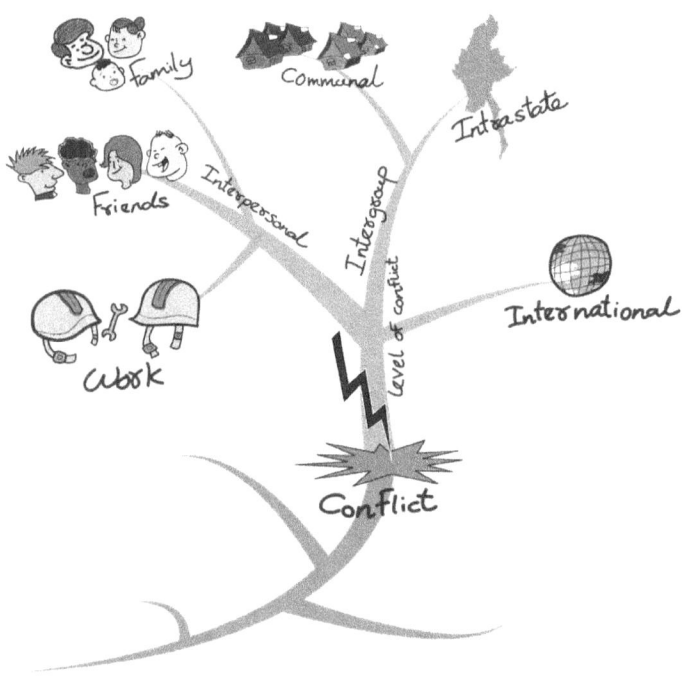

Using Mind Maps

Using mind maps does not need to be that intimidating. You simply follow a handful of steps accordingly.
By following these steps, you will find that your map will naturally come together.

Keep in mind that there is software that you can use to make mind maps on your computer or phone, or you can choose to do so the old fashioned way, on paper with a pen or pencil.
No matter how you choose to do so, however, you should get a pretty similar end result either way, and it will look something like this:

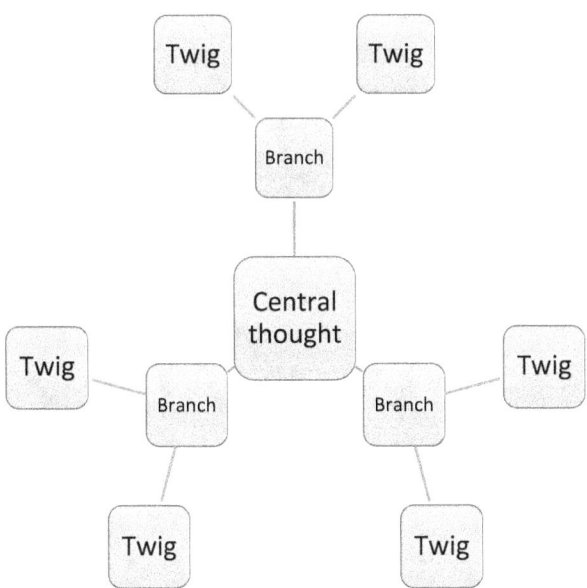

Of course, you will be free to add in all of the shapes, colors, images, and anything else that you think is relevant to the formation of your map, and you are free to work in any order that you want.

You can have your central thought in the middle of the page with branches all around it, like a tree from an aerial view, or you can do so in any other way that makes the most sense to you.

1. Identify your main theme:

You will start the process by first figuring out what your main theme of your map will be. Let's consider what it would look like if you were, for example, trying to figure out how to address your toddler's stubborn eating problem. Perhaps your toddler refuses to eat, and so you write down, "Foods Liam will eat."

> Foods
> Liam
> will eat

2. Identify your subthemes:

Now, it is time to start figuring out any of the relevant categories that you need to make. You then would start to branch out from that initial central thought. In this case, perhaps you start with food groups so you can plan out all of the food groups your toddler should be regularly eating. Note how the subthemes are short—each one is only a single word long. This means that you have more space on your sheet for other information, and you are getting the basics down at the same time.

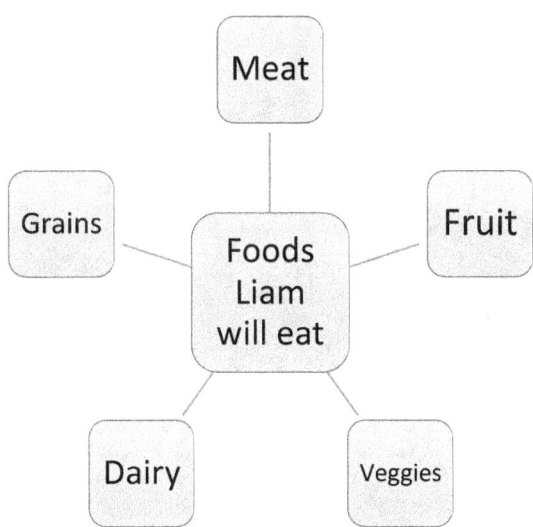

3. Add your twigs to the branches:

Now, you need to start figuring out everything that you are going to write on those branches. Your branches should each get at least two or three twigs per branch, and they will help you further your planning. Notice how the mind map begins to grow in size quite quickly. You can continue to use words, phrases, and images as you see fit. At the end of making the mind map, now, you can look all around the perimeter at a nice and neat list for your child's food preferences.

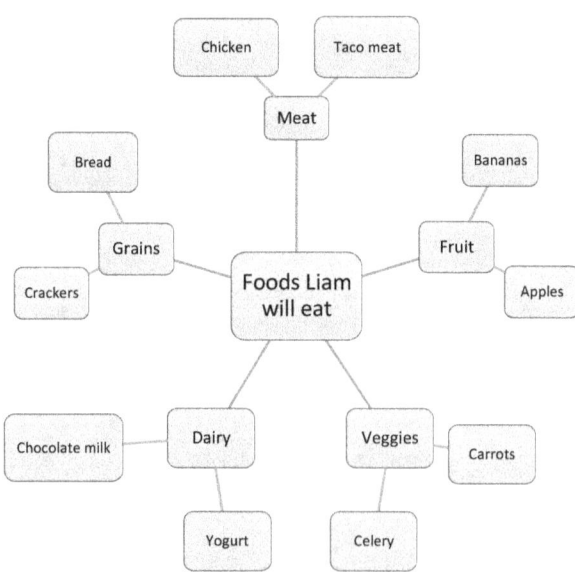

At the end of the day, you can use mind mapping for just about anything.

You can use it to figure out your main characters for a novel, or to figure out what you need to do before you move.

You can use it to sort out your thoughts in order to get a clearer idea of what is going on in your mind, or you can use it just to try to organize yourself.

No matter what, however, having all of the information all laid out in front of you in easily referenceable forms means that you will be able to track your thoughts with ease.

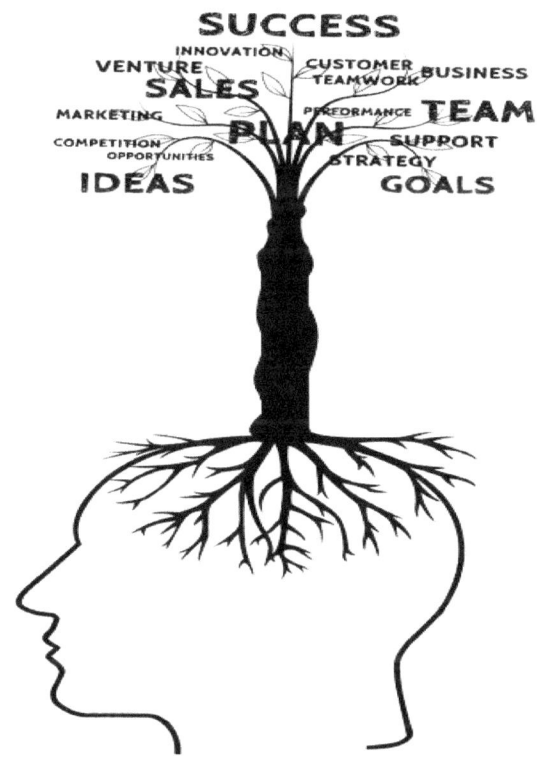

Chapter 7: The Body and Remembering

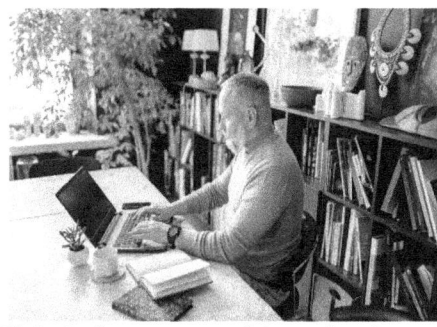

Some people happen to find that they learn best when they use their bodies as cues. When they are able to use their bodies, they find that learning becomes so much easier.

This is known as kinesthetic memory. You may recognize this with children in particular: They learn best when they are actively running around and playing, and sitting them down can actually interfere with their learning.

Think about how children learn nursery rhymes when they are young—they learn through movement. There is the song, for example,

The Itsy Bitsy Spider and the hand motions that go along with it—the children learn them in tandem, and they can use the words to remind them of the hand movements and vice versa.

While some people eventually move on to different kinds of preferences for memory making, others still find that they are best able to remember when they can come up with some sort of movement to go along with it.

You may be amongst those kinesthetic memory people, and that is okay. At the end of the day, so long as you are able to remember, that is all that matters. Now, let's delve into kinesthetic memory, how it works, and how to use it.

The Body and Memory

Kinesthetic learning can become quite difficult to use as you move into adulthood.
While it may have been cute to watch a bunch of kids act out, Heads, Shoulders, Knees, and Toes at their preschool concert, it is not quite so endearing when you see an adult walking around and miming the instructions to their next work assignment.
If you saw someone standing there, moving his hands left and right as he thought out the directions to get to the nearest gas station in an unfamiliar area in town after asking for help, you might think he or she was crazy — after all, why else would he be flopping his hands about like a fish?

Despite the fact that the world is not built for kinesthetic learners, it is still incredibly valid and useful. People everywhere find that they are able to actively use these methods to help them remember.
They may find that doodling becomes a way of helping them focus, allowing them to move somehow. Others may find that they can simply tap their feet or fingers as they listen. Others still may find that the building of a diagram or actively seeking out a way to take apart something that they are learning about, that active doing of the activity can help them actually learn it.

There is nothing wrong with this if it works for you — if you are going to remember what you are learning simply by tapping your toes to a certain rhythm, perhaps the rhythm of the syllables, or in dipping your head one way or the other, you should take advantage.

The Senses and Memory

You may have heard, at one point or another, that playing music or chewing gum when learning something can help you remember it again in the future if you can create the same sort of sensory input.

This is true—you create those associations, and it has been proven that people can better remember things when they are in the same state in which they learned them in the first place.

If you want to chew mint gum while studying for your math test, or when you are learning all of those important rules for work, go for it—so long as you are going to be able to chew that gum again any other time you need to remember that information.

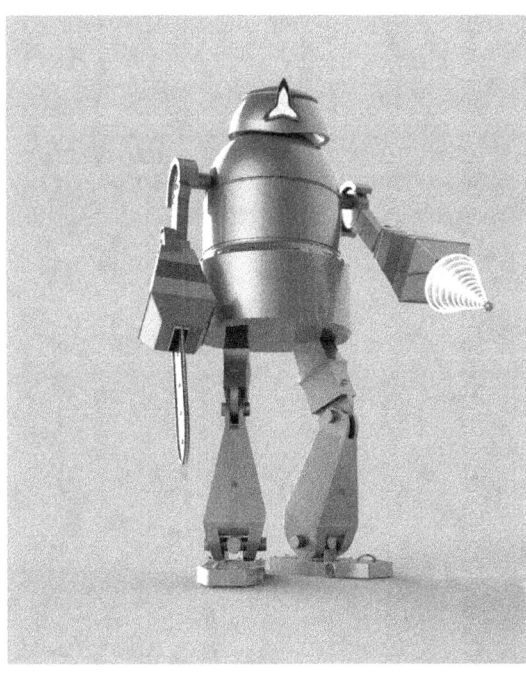

Your senses work well to help you remember simply because the more sense that you can add to the situation, the more likely you are to properly encode it all.

Think about it this way—you may hear something said to you, such as if you were being lectured. That is great, but

83

are you likely to remember it in particular? Not necessarily on its own—you need other sensory stimulation to strengthen those connections.

This is why so often, teachers and professors will actively use slideshows or other visual stimuli as they lecture—it is more effective if the information is being registered in more ways than one.

This means, then, that engaging more than one sense is the perfect way to remember something.

Instead of silently reading over that phone number that you need to remember, try saying it out loud to yourself as you read it. Now, you are actively stating the information, you hear yourself say it out loud, and you are reading it at the same time.

For even more effect, you could try layering it even more with your hands, feeling the numbers by actively flashing them. After each number, hold up the appropriate number of fingers.

Effectively, the more involved you make your body and senses in trying to encode the memory, the more likely you are to actually remember it in the future.

Using the Body and Memory

Using your body to remember does not need to be difficult—you can do it in all sorts of different ways.

All that is important is that you are actively engaging with the information and moving your body at the same time.

Not only does this heighten your awareness and arousal simply because you are being active, but you also create more pathways for your brain to remember the information, and that alone can have a massive impact on how well you will remember what is in front of you.

All you need to do to boost your memory then is to figure out how to pair that information with some sort of movement or sensation.

If you sing the words that you need to remember, you make it easier for you to remember in the future, especially if you do it to the sound of a song that you already know.

You could make a timeline that you write down across a room, and slowly walk along the line as you go over the information in your mind.

Really, the options are endless, so long as you get up and involve your body somehow.

Clenching Fists to Concentrate and Remember

Some people find that clenching the fists for brief periods of time can actually increase brain activity.

In particular, when you clench your left fist, you activate the right prefrontal area in your brain, which is responsible for remembering things.

On the other hand, clenching your right fist triggers activation in the left prefrontal area, which is responsible for encoding memory.

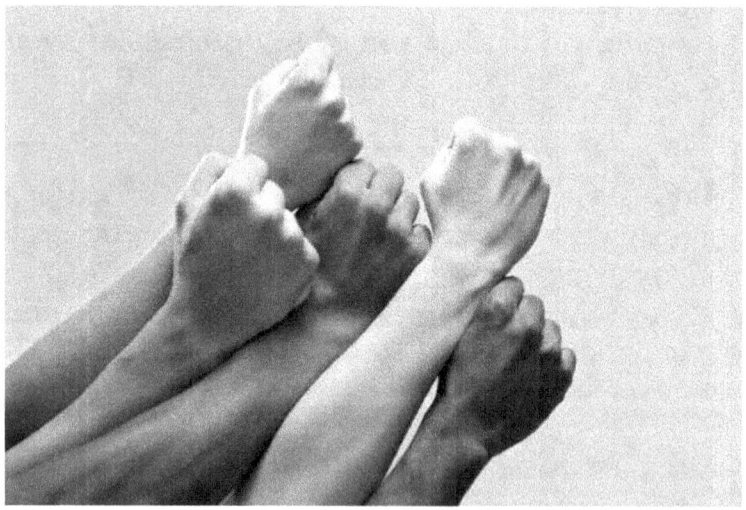

This means, then, that you can increase brain activity in the appropriate area when you need to either encode or remember information.

In particular, when you are learning material, you should clench your right fist for 90 seconds before reading over it. You give your brain a boost to help it encode that information into the right places.

Then, when you want to remember the information, you can then clench your left fist for 90 seconds to help your mind work more effectively.

Keep in mind; if you are left-handed, you will need to do the opposite. However, it still works the same way—you can clench your fist to help encode the memory for learning, and then you can clench the other fist in order to recall it.

Left-handed People	Right-handed People
• Clench left hand into a fist for 90 seconds • Learn • Right before recall, clench right fist for 90 seconds • Recall the information	• Clench right hand into fist for 90 seconds • Learn • Right before recall, clench left fist for 90 seconds • Recall the information

Moving Eyes From Side to Side to Improve Learning

Another interesting trick to use your body to better learn and focus is through moving your eyes. In particular, you must move your eyes from side to side rather than up and down.

This is because you are making both sides of the brain communicate when you move your eyes horizontally, and this allows you to better recall memories. This may look somewhat silly in practice, but the usefulness of it is undeniable.

All you need to do is remember to move your eyes back and forth, from side to side, for 30 seconds before you try to learn something.

If you are trying to remember a list, for example, you may dart your eyes from side to side for 30 seconds and then read over it. Then, when you need to recall the information later on, you can move your eyes back and forth again as you try to remember it, perhaps at the store when you are making your purchases.

Moving eyes horizontally for memory

- Move eyes back and forth horizontally for 30 seconds
- Learn new material
- Move eyes again when you are struggling to recall

Practical Exercises to Train the Brain

Now, at this point, you have a pretty good idea of several ways that you can boost learning and train your brain. However, there are other ways that you can increase your ability to recall information as well.

You may find that sometimes, you need to remember that list of information. Others, you need to remember a name of someone that you have not talked to in ages.

No matter the situation or what you need to do, it can be embarrassing when you struggle to get something right. For that reason, you may choose to strengthen your brain and help yourself remember better before that issue of forgetting comes up in the first place. Within this section of the book, we are going to go over techniques for several situations that can help you. We will take a look at:

- How to remember names and faces
- How to remember numbers and data
- How to remember directions
- How to remember lists
- How to use creativity to remember
- How to use calculations
- How to speed read
- What to eat to help with memory
- How to exercise to help with memor

Remembering Names and Faces

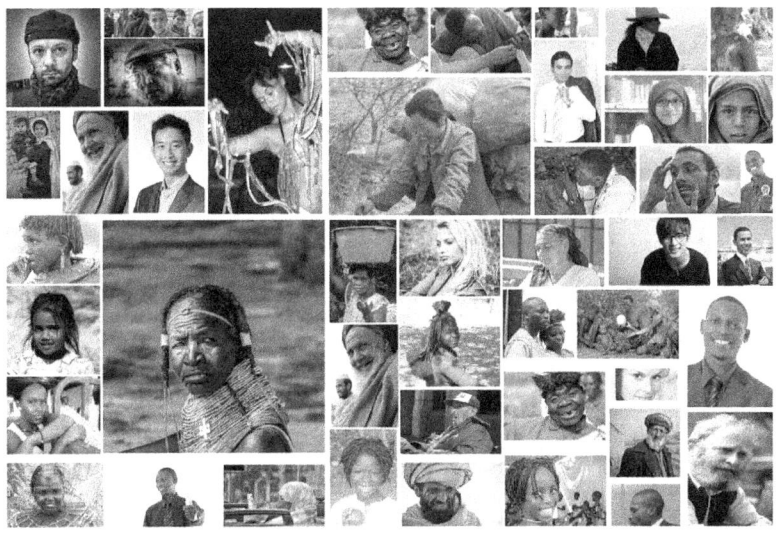

No one wants to be in that situation where they forget to remember the name of someone important, or forget which face goes along with whose name. Yet, this happens all the time.

Spare yourself the embarrassment and try one of these tips to help you remember names and faces.

Remind yourself of your motivator

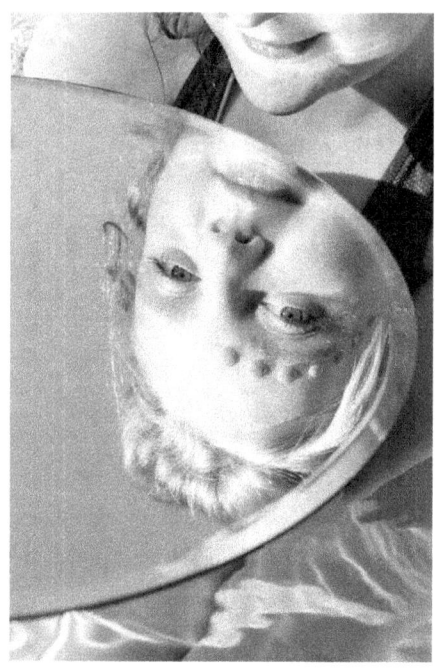

If you know that this name and face is important, remind yourself of what is on the hook if you fail to remember it. Is this the name of your new boss or the person that interviewed you? Is it the name of someone who will be relevant to you later on?

Perhaps he is a client that you are trying to win over, and you need to make sure that you get his name right so you do not blow your deal.

When you make sure that you know what is motivating you to remember their name, suddenly, you make their name and face seem that much more valuable to your brain.

If you do not have a particular reason that you want to learn their name other than liking them or wanting to be polite, up the ante—tell yourself that your life depends upon your ability to remember this person's name tomorrow—and then try to remember it.

Link the name to a prominent feature

Everyone has something about them that is distinctive in some way, even if what is distinctive is that they are so plain looking or average, and that is okay.
However, you can take advantage of this—all you need to do is make sure that you are actively thinking of their name and pair it to a name.
Instead of John, they become John with the bright green eyes, or instead of Freya, you have Freya with the wildly curly hair.
This helps you figure out how to identify each name and face and makes both just a bit more memorable for you in the future.
When you have something else to fall back upon, remembering the name becomes just a bit easier.

Repeat their name back to them when you part

One final way that may help is that if you are actively trying to remember a new name, when you and the other person part, make sure that you end your greeting with their name. Instead of saying, "Okay, bye!" you could try, "It was great meeting you, Freya," or, "Thanks for taking the time to talk to me, John!" Just using their name helps you push it further and further into your memory for future use.

Remembering Numbers and Data

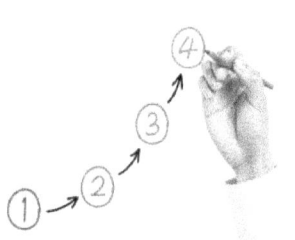
Numbers, like names, seem to be everywhere. When you have to enter PINs and passwords with number sequences that are not 1234, you may find that it is difficult to keep track of them all. Especially since numbers are abstract, they become difficult to remember.

While you might be able to remember 5 onions, because you know that onions are not abstract, you may struggle to recall the number 52463 or some other series of number that is arbitrary, such as a phone number, a ZIP code, a PIN, or a credit card number.

This is where these techniques come in. With the help of these techniques, you will be able to remember longer strands of numbers, even if they seem to be meaningless.

Consider the number as if it were being typed on a number pad

While number pads are quickly going obsolete, you can still find them in areas such as on your phone's lock screen if you use a PIN. Look at how the number strand that you are trying to remember lines up with that number pad. 75391 looks like an X shape if you were to type it in on a number pad, or 85264 would look like a +.

It can also help if you tap out that pattern if it is not something that you can easily identify. You can actively recall the pattern to yourself for a longer strand of numbers if you repeat it to yourself enough.

Create an association with the number

Another way that you can help yourself remember those number strands is through figuring out how best to break numbers up into patterns you can associate with something else. If, for example, you need to remember the phone number 342-9192 you may start by breaking it down to something you can remember—On March 3, your 4th child turned 2.
You and your partner were born in 1991 and 1992. Suddenly, you have a way to remember that number because you made it relevant to yourself. You tell yourself that the number is the day your fourth child turned two, and the years of your and your husband's birth.

You may find that you need other associations as well. Perhaps it is the number of your favorite baseball player, or your address.
Maybe it is the name of a song, or the date or age that you did something significant.
No matter what, however, if you can make the numbers lose their arbitrariness that they had that made things difficult in the first place, you can start to figure out how best to recall them in the future.

Break the number down into smaller bits

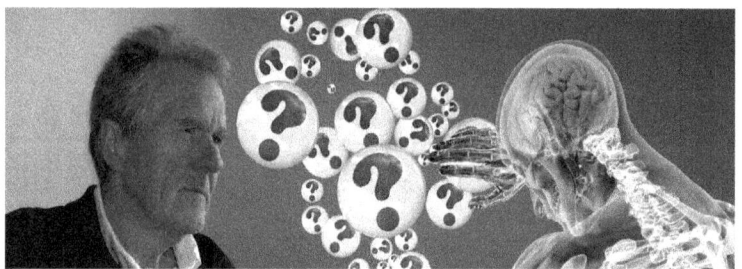

Sometimes, it is simply too hard to remember all of the numbers in a long sequence. After all, if you were told to remember 98325157, would you be able to? At first glance, probably not.
However, if you were to break it down into smaller, more manageable parts, you would probably be able to.
For example, if instead of remembering 98325157, you were told to remember 983, 251, and 57, you probably could. This is because you are now using smaller numbers that are far more manageable.
This is a great way to remember phone numbers as well — you can break them down into smaller bits.

Instead of having 3038328391, a random phone number, to remember and being overwhelmed, you can break it up with pauses in your memory and in your repetition.
It becomes 303-832-8391. Now, you can break this down even further — 303, 832, 83, 91. You kind of hear this sort of inflection when you recite phone numbers as well — you sort of pause naturally after the third, sixth, and eighth number when someone is writing the number down, and if you remember to pause your own recollection of the

numbers at those points as well, you may find that remembering becomes far easier.

Remembering Directions

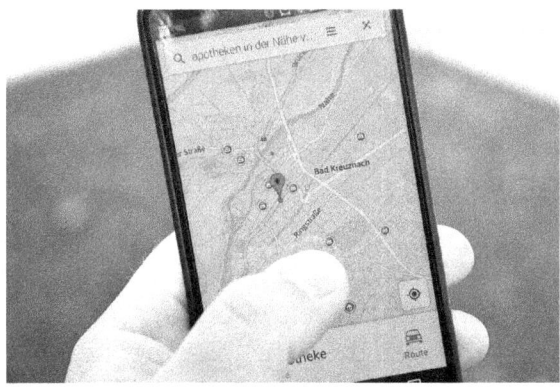

Now, admittedly, very rarely do people actually have to remember directions these days. You have GPS ready for you in nearly any situation, but what if your phone died? If you had literally no way to get online to use GPS to guide you, would you be able to remember some simple directions?

Now, you can be prepared with these techniques.

Associate an image with left and right

Perhaps one of the most difficult parts of remembering directions is remembering if you were supposed to go left or right on any given street.

Obviously, going the wrong direction is going to land you in somewhere far different than you were hoping to get to, so being able to navigate accordingly becomes incredibly important.

An easy way to remember left or right is to give each its own association. Perhaps you choose to remember lizards when you need to turn left, and runners when you need to turn right. When you know that you need to turn left on Main ST., you should remind yourself that there are lizards on Main St. Picture lizards literally sitting on the street, and you will remember left.

Likewise, you can choose to imagine runners going down instead if you need to turn right.

Repeat them back

Of course, this seems like common sense, but if, when you first ask for directions and get them from someone, you actively repeat them back to the other person to hear, you are more likely to remember it.

However, there is no rule that you cannot keep going. In fact, you should keep going.

Continue the process by telling yourself over and over again how to get there. Repeat to yourself every few minutes that you are going to turn left on Main ST, then turn right on 4th Ave, and finally turning left again on Oak St. It will be easier to remember the more you recite it.

Turn it into a story

This may be more useful for a longer strand of directions, but you may be able to turn the street directions into a story for yourself.

Of course, it is likely to be quite a short story, but you will still be able to take advantage of it.

For example, you may tell yourself in this instance that the MAIN thing that you are looking forward to on the FOURTH of July is sitting under that big OAK tree in your backyard so you can watch the fireworks.

Suddenly, instead of arbitrary names of city streets, you have a short story that you can repeat to yourself to remind you of which streets are important and which you can ignore.

Of course, you may need to get creative with this, and sometimes, you may find that you need more than just a story.

After all, can you really make a story out of a series of numbered street names? It might get kind of difficult.

Create landmarks and associations

What may also help you as you go through trying to remember those directions is figuring out if there are any landmarks to keep track of.

Instead of worrying about which street to turn onto, maybe consider instead whether you can use other visual landmarks that are a bit less arbitrary.

Perhaps you turn left at the Starbucks next to the pizzeria, and then you turn right next to that bench with the tree over it, two blocks down. In making other sorts of ways that you can remember what is around you, you may find that it is actually easier to remember.

After all, painting a picture is oftentimes far easier to remember than trying to remember the names of streets that will not have any sort of picture for you to think about unless you make one for yourself.

Remembering Shopping Lists

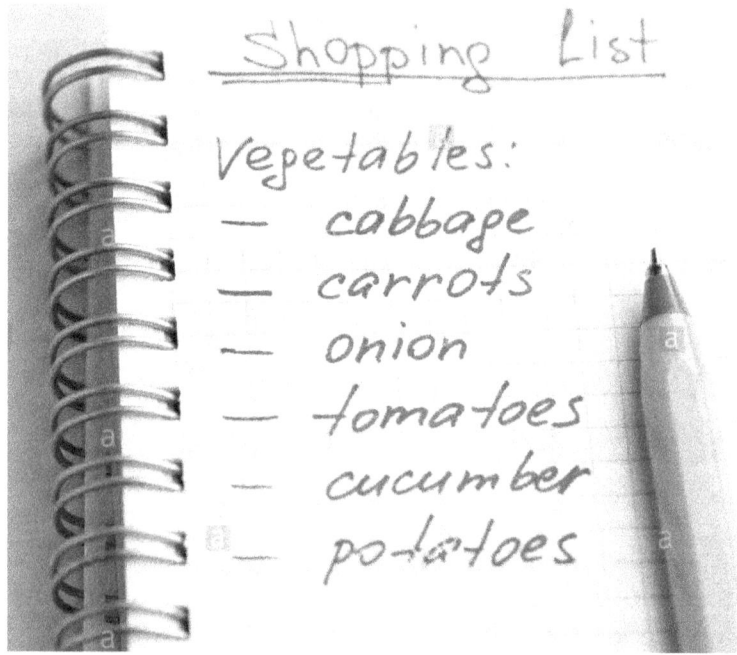

Everyone has been there before—you made a shopping list, but you cannot remember what was on it.
This is incredibly frustrating, especially if you have quite a drive back home to reclaim the list. Y
ou try your best to get everything on the list, but it feels like there is always at least a handful of things that are forgotten, and for some reason, those forgotten items are always the most important ones on the list.
You can put an end to this by memorizing your shopping lists instead, especially if they are on the shorter side.

Write your list in a silly font

Interestingly enough, when you read something in a fond that is somewhat tricky to discern, it becomes easier to remember.

There is a reason for this—when you use a silly font to write out your list and then read over it, your brain has to work harder to read it.

This makes it more memorable because you broke up the fluency with which you read it. Because your brain works harder, you then store the memory in a way that is more concrete—it becomes a stronger memory for the time being.

This effect works with all sorts of lists or written material. If you need to memorize written material, make it difficult to read, but still legible, and you will be more likely to remember it later.

For example, imagine how difficult it would be to read a widely looping font as opposed to the straightforward font that you see in most books—your reading speed would be dropped dramatically until your brain adjusted accordingly.

You would also be more likely to recall anything that you read more easily as well, however.

Use a memory palace

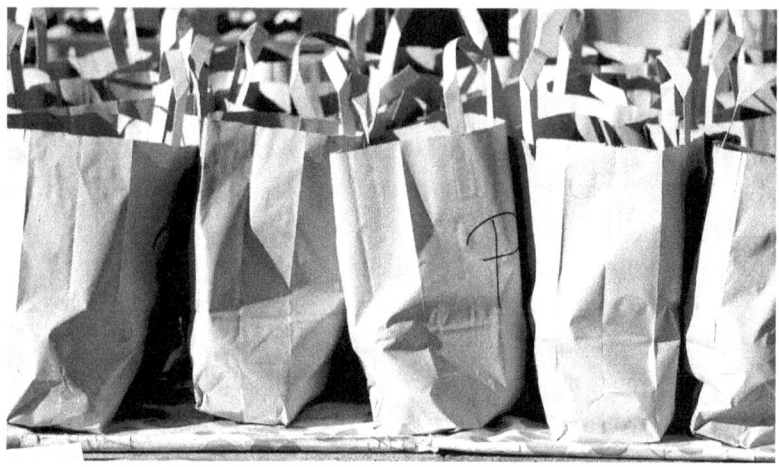

This technique may seem a bit strange, especially if you will be using a shopping list for food, however, bear with it for a moment and see if it works for you.

Think about the most common route you take through your home.

Perhaps it is the path from your bedroom to the kitchen since you will be cooking food in the kitchen.

Along the way, you pass the following rooms:

1. Master bedroom
2. Child's bedroom
3. Bathroom
4. Laundry room
5. Hallway
6. Staircase
7. Living room
8. Dining room
9. Kitchen

10. Refrigerator

Now, you always walk past all of those rooms as you go to the fridge to get the ingredients out for dinner.

You will now pair up the ten items on your list with these locations. Perhaps you are buying

1. Milk
2. Eggs
3. Bread
4. Chicken
5. Rice
6. Apples
7. Carrots
8. Bell pepper
9. Pizza
10. Ice cream

Now, you must match up each of those items to a room in your house on your journey.

When you are trying to memorize your shopping list, you would think about milk being in your bedroom, and eggs in your child's room. You would go down the list, room to room until you found ice cream in the refrigerator.

By matching up each room with a different item, and then following that journey through your mind when you are at the store, you can better remember your items.

You may remember that bottle of milk on your bed and wonder why it is there, or point out to yourself how absurd it was that ice cream was in the fridge.

At the end of the day, however, you are likely to better remember your list.

Create nonsense acronyms

If, at the end of the day, what you need is memorable, what is more memorable than something that sounds ridiculous? If you have children, you may be able to turn it into a game — who can make the most ridiculous sounding acronym with the shopping list to make sure that it is memorable? Your children's abilities may surprise you.

Let's take our list again:

1. Milk
2. Eggs
3. Bread
4. Chicken
5. Rice
6. Apples
7. Carrots
8. Bell pepper
9. Pizza
10. Ice cream

It is already set up for a few natural acronyms: MEB and CRAC, being two that stand out. So, what if you swapped pizza and ice cream? Now, you have MEB, CRAC, BIP. Your children may have fun pretending to be a robot as they walk through the grocery store, uttering those words, or you are left wondering what is left of your sanity as you do so yourself.

Either way, you suddenly have something silly and smaller that you can break down. You need to buy MEB? Okay — you know you can break it down into milk, eggs, and bread. CRAC? You needed chicken, rice, apples, and carrots. BIP—you needed bell peppers, ice cream, and pizza.

The more ridiculous and memorable something is, the easier it will be to remember at the end of the day. Use that to your advantage.

Using Creativity

Creativity is, in essence, a form of intelligence and memory. You can use your creativity to remember things better. Consider most of the methods for remembering things that have been brought up thus far? T
hey have been creative—you have been making new words or visualizing ridiculous situations in order to remember something new, and for good reason.

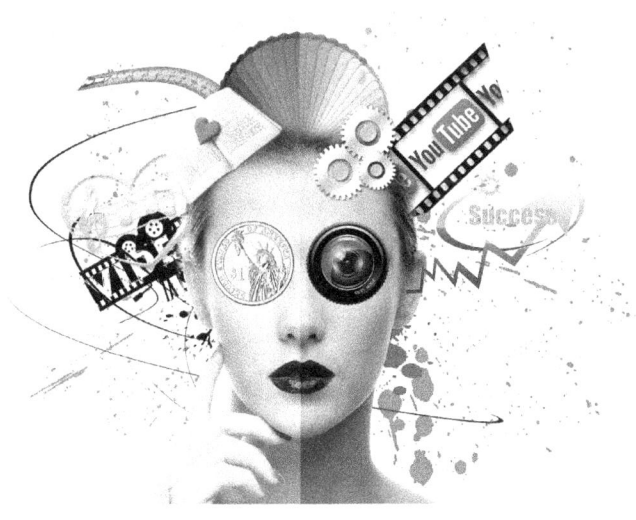

When you are being creative, you are engaging in divergent thinking—you are exploring many different options and possibilities and choosing out the best possible one.

In being creative, you are actively thinking about things in a different way, and this means that your brain is having to make more pathways, use more information, and figure out other ways to use something, all of which will help push the point of improving memory.

Think about all the ways that you can use a safety pin; for example—you may say that you can use it to attach clothing together, for example.

Is that particularly creative? Not really.

However, if you said that you wanted to use the safety pins and clip them all together to make chainmail armor, that is a lot more unexpected. That is creative thinking.

Those who are more creative, who do come up with these off-the-wall suggestions, tend to find that they can remember better than those who do not. The reason for this may surprise you; however—creativity requires high memory.

In order to be creative, you must be able to remember things. For example, if you are going to be making something memorable, you need to make it seem crazy or creative. This is easy enough to understand.

How, then, can you use creativity to boost your own memory and train your brain? There are actually several ways in which you can do just that.

Repeating things back to yourself—but in different words

One way to utilize your creativity is through actively repeating things back to yourself, but putting a new spin on them. Perhaps you, for example, make it a point to actively explain something back to yourself in a different manner.

By being able to rephrase something rather than just parrot it back to yourself, you are making it clear that you actually understand what you are talking about in the first place, and this means that you are more likely to remember it in the future.

For example, perhaps you need to remember a list of items for your dinner party—you can remember them by reciting the recipe to yourself in different words than you had initially read them in.

For example, maybe you mention to yourself, that you need to sauté the onion and garlic, then braise the meat, and then finally, use a splash of wine to deglaze the pan. You tell yourself all of this, not necessarily paying attention to the exact amounts of ingredients, but also actively making sure that you understand them.

You also have the added benefit of reinforcing that you need to buy onions, garlic, meat, and wine for that recipe.

Let your imagination run free

Sometimes, it can help you to remember something if you let your mind run wild. For example, if you just learned something new, such as that pineapples do not, in fact, grow on trees, you may imagine crazy little bushes where giant pineapples are hanging out.

In making it as silly as possible for yourself to remember, you will find that it is far more memorable than it otherwise would have been.

As an added bonus, you also strengthen your own ability to remember things better in the future! You flex those creative muscles, meaning that you are able to better utilize them the next time that you need them.

Calculation

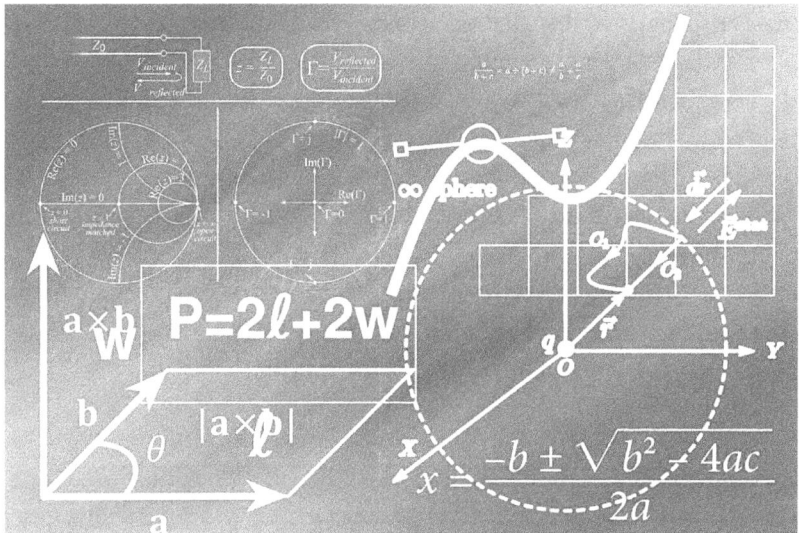

You may look at this section and realize that these days, being able to do mental calculations is practically completely obsolete, and it is.
However, you can still see all sorts of important benefits from being able to run calculations on your own.
Now, your math teacher may have been wrong about saying that you will not always have a calculator in your pocket—most of us do now in the form of cell phones. However, that does not mean that learning how to run calculations is entirely useless for your brain.

Think of it this way—you have a car now, so needing to walk or run long distances is pointless. However, it is still good for you to walk and run sometimes — it is good for your body.

In this instance, your running of calculations is working mental muscles that would otherwise have gone neglected.

In particular, when you are doing mental calculations, you are going to be doing math without any aids at all — no calculators, and no paper or pencil.

It is commonly done for sport and competition these days rather than actually being required, but it can still help you strengthen your mind.

There are major benefits to having a sharp mind, such as being able to think quicker and with more rationality.

While this may be difficult at first, you will be able to actively run mental math far better than before after practicing with the following techniques.

Replacing subtracting with addition

When people are asked to add numbers together, they seem to have no issues doing so — it is quite straightforward. However, subtracting seems to be far more difficult for some strange reason.

Instead of struggling with the subtraction, however, you can actively go with addition instead.

For example, imagine that you need to make three stops at three different stores.

You only have $200 on you to get through all three stores, and you need to do a stock up on groceries, make sure that you have money to buy pet supplies at the pet store, and also make sure that you stop to get paper products at your local retailer.

You know that dog food will cost you $32, and that the paper products cost you $29. You need to know how much money you have available to buy groceries at the store. You know that the dog food and paper products together cost you $61.
How much money is then spendable to you at the grocery store so you can comfortably buy everything?

Now, you may struggle with straight subtraction, but you can ask yourself, instead, how much do you have to add to 61 to get to 200? Switching the context can sometimes help with mental math.
Now, all you do is add 9 to 61 to get 70, and then you know that 70 needs 130 more to get to 200. From there, 130 + 9 is 139, so you have $139 available.

Of course, that was a very simple example of when you may need to use addition instead of subtraction.
When you are dealing with larger or more complex numbers, such as 8312 – 5324, you may find that figuring out what you have to add to 5324 is easier than trying to mentally subtract it.

Multiply in parts instead of as a whole

Another tricky calculation can be multiplication for larger numbers, especially if they are beyond the times table that you were forced to memorize early on in school.
 In these situations, you may find that it is far easier to break up what you are multiplying and add it up instead.

For example, imagine that you need to multiply 7 x 23. This is not a very round number by any means—but you can break it up.
Instead, you can multiply 7 x 20 and 7 x 3 and then add them together.

In this instance, then, you would get
7 x 20 = 140
7 x 3 = 21
21 + 140 = 161

Quickly entering that into your calculator tells you that 7 x 23 is, in fact, 161. Now you can tackle those more complex multiplication problems in your head a bit easier! Of course, the more you practice, the easier this will all become. These skills and mental calculations are effectively just muscles that you need to practice.
The more you practice them, the stronger it will become.

Multiplying by 4 or 8 just requires you to double numbers

When you have to multiply by 2, you are probably pretty quick to do so.

However, when that becomes multiplying by 4 or 8, you may find that you are intimidated. Instead, focus on the fact that 4 is just multiplying by 2 twice, and 8 is then multiplying by 2 three times over. So, if you want to get 4 x 37, for example, you would just double 37 to get 74, and then double 74 to get 148.

Likewise, if you wanted 8 x 37, you would then double 148 as well to get 296.

This can help with all sorts of math if you need to run it, or can at least be a quick game that you play to strengthen your own mind.

You could try racing yourself—how many times can you double a number before it gets too big for you to mess with in your mind?

Speed Reading

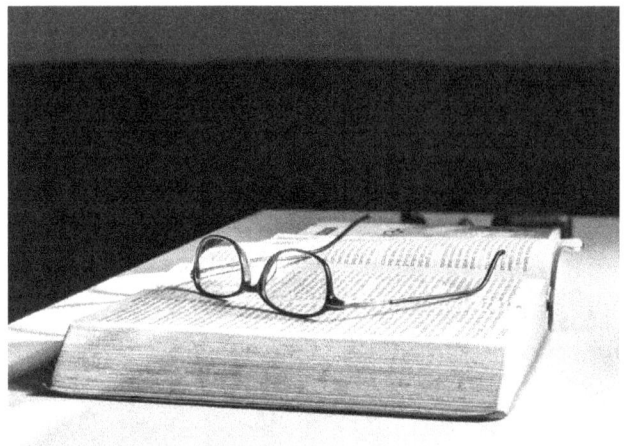

Speed reading is something that everyone wishes they had—if you can read quickly, you can save time, and in this day and age, who couldn't use some time to save? Everyone wants to get that extra bit of time to themselves, or spent with their friends or family, and if you have a job that requires extensive reading, you may find that you can cut down the time that you spend doing it through learning to speed read.

So much of our lives are spent reading—you are reading this as we go! You may read on social media, or read the news to understand what is happening in the world around you.

People tend to read at roughly 250 words per minute when they are trying to comprehend it.

However, there are ways to up this speed. What would you do if you could spend half of the time that you currently spend reading doing something else? What would you want to do with that time?

First, let's consider when speed reading is a good idea to use—it is helpful to read quicker, but you need to keep in mind that there is a degree to which reading quickly will also lessen your comprehension.

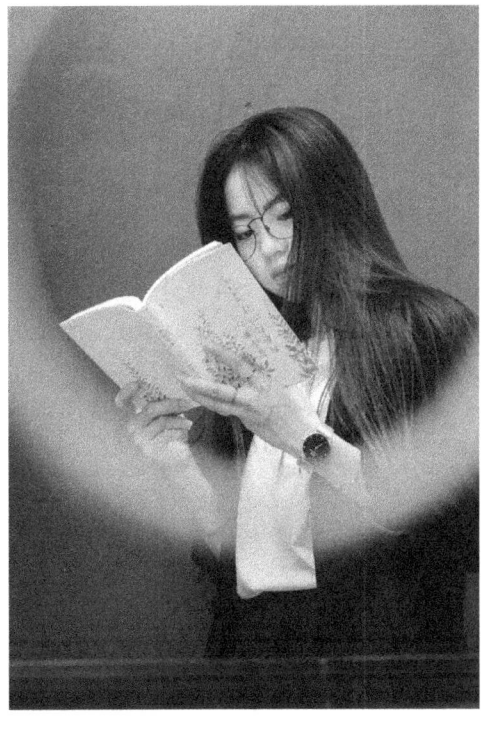

If you need a vague idea of what you are addressing, then yes, speed reading may be good for you.

However, if you are going to have a test soon on all of the information, then it may be better for you to instead slow down and focus on the words in detail.

A lawyer, for example, probably wants to read through everything word for word, as many legal documents are going to be incredibly specific and thorough. Reading through the news on your lunch break, however, is not necessarily quite as important to do in detail.

As a general rule, when you want to memorize something, you need to read it slowly, usually right around or below 100 words per minute.

However, if you are learning, you will read around 100-200 words per minute, and just comprehending is anywhere from 200-400 words per minute.

This then implies that any reading that you are doing above 500 words per minute is going to be sacrificing some degree of comprehension, so you need to weigh if the document that you are reading is right to speed read.

When most people read, they do so by saying the words in their minds. They see the word, "Pizza," and they say the word in their mind.

However, when you speed read, you stop that from happening. Instead of uttering the word in your mind, you skim over the words—you are then able to effectively comprehend the word without pronouncing the world, and this ups your ability to read quicker.

This can be difficult for people to do—after all, you probably learned to read out loud at first, and eventually moved that internal.

Most people do read to themselves, but if you want to actively avoid pronouncing them, you can do so by forcing yourself to relax.

You will start this process by learning to relax your face and allow your gaze to focus on more than one word at a time—you stop seeing words as individual words and instead see them as strings of words, which allows you to skip across the page quicker than before.

As you arrive at the end of a line, you allow your peripheral vision to move your eye to read the next line while reading those words with your peripheral vision instead.

You then skip the line quickly while still processing the words that came before that point.

There are several methods through which you can do this—you can make it a point to point and read, or track and pace. We will go over the three most common methods of speed reading for you now.

The pointer method

This is a method through which you use your hand or a fingertip to point at the words as you go and guide yourself along the words.

Effectively, you sweep your finger over the words as you read, and you are able to do so far quicker than if you were just letting your eyes go about it.

It effectively sharpens your ability to focus on the words in front of you, and this means that your speed can then improve.

The track and pace method

This is quite similar to the pointer method, but in this case, you are going to be using a pen as you read instead. With the cap on the pen, point it under the word that you are going to start at, and then drag the pen across the words rapidly.

Your eyes will follow just above where the pen touches the paper and will increase your focus on the words. This will allow you to again focus while moving quicker than you otherwise would have.

Make it a point to spend no more than a single second on each line that you are reading.

Over time, you will see your speed increase. Your brain will catch on to what you are doing and adapt accordingly, allowing you to further make use of this method.

The scanning method

Finally, let's consider the scanning method. This is perhaps the least thorough of all, but it is also the quickest.

When you are scanning, you are effectively just running down the center of the page, reading the information, and picking up on key words or phrases.

You may pick up key sentences, such as the first sentences in paragraphs, or anything bolded. You may also pick up actions and names or dates.

While you will not get everything in this method all at once, you will actively get all sorts of background and preliminary information that you can use to get the basic concept down.

With enough practice, you will find that any of these methods would get easier.

Your brain just needs the practice, and the more you actively train it, the more likely you are to actively learn how to do what you set out to do.

If you want to be able to read 1000 words per minute, then more power to you! All you need to do is stick to the program and continue to practice.

When you want to improve your speed reading, it becomes important for you to keep a few key points in mind.

You want to make sure that you are not distracted when you are trying to speed read—you need to focus on the words in front of you as much as humanly possible, and you cannot do that if you are in a noisy or otherwise non-conducive environment.

You need your setting to be relaxed.

You may also find that starting easy is a good way to go—don't break out the Shakespeare and expect to actually absorb anything if you start speed reading.

Start with some simpler books or things that you find enjoyable—novels or other light reading would be a great place to begin.

Test yourself as you go to make sure that you are, in fact, absorbing information.

Finally, you may also find benefit in tracking your speeds as they improve. Over time, you may realize that you improved far more than you thought was possible and be shocked to discover that you did, in fact, drastically improve your speed when you thought you had already plateaued.

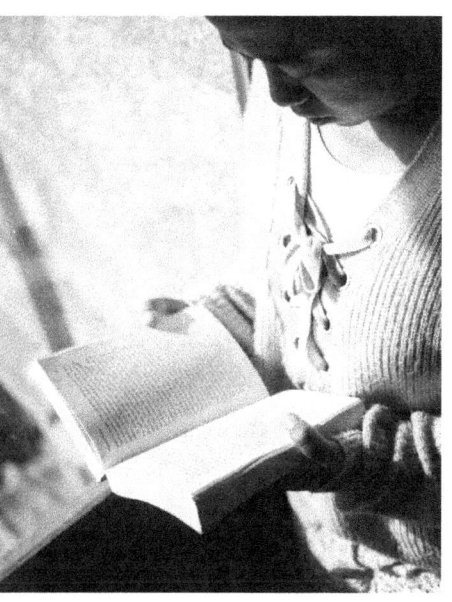

There are all sorts of programs and trackers online that can help with this.

Brain Food

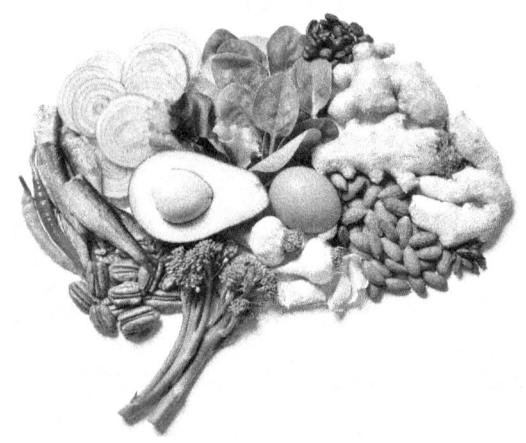

You are what you eat, and your brain is no exception to that. If you eat poorly, you are going to find that your entire body seems to drag on and struggle.

You may not have the energy that you need to move on in your day, or you may feel like you are foggy or unable to think.

This is not for nothing—your brain is incredibly complex, and it has very specific needs. If you are not meeting those needs, you are going to find that you struggle to ever actually live as healthily as you should be.

Of course, if you are what you eat, then you should also be able to improve your body's function by making sure that you are eating healthily.

By making sure that you eat food that is good brain fuel, you will find that your own ability to comprehend what you are doing will increase exponentially.

Your ability to think will seem so much easier if you are not bogged down by sugar hazes or otherwise feeling ill. Eating for your brain does not have to be particularly unenjoyable either—there are plenty of delicious foods that will deliver that nutritious punch that your body needs.

Fatty fish

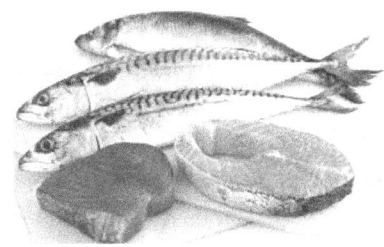

Most people already assume that salmon is brain fuel and for good reason. It is full of omega-3 fatty acids, and because your brain is made primarily of fat, it needs fat to help maintain itself.

Your brain will make great use of all of those fatty acids in these fish, allowing it to repair brain and nerve cells. In repairing those cells, you will find that your brain is also able to boost memory and learning.

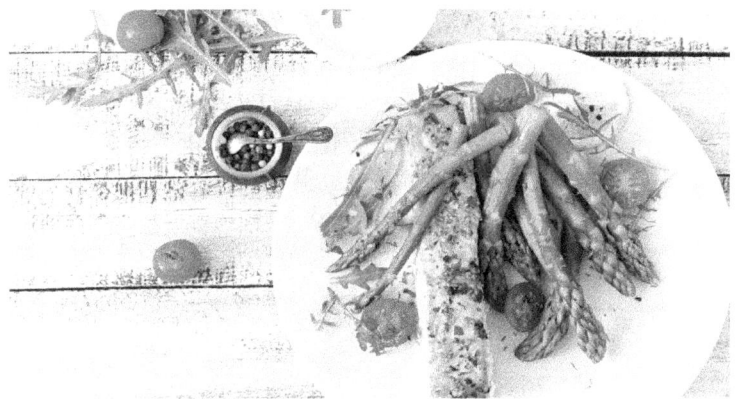

Not only that, but eating fatty fish can help with avoiding age-related struggling to think clearly and helps fend off the development of Alzheimer's disease.

Without enough of these omega-3s, however, you may find that you struggle.

Overall, it has been shown that those who eat fish regularly have more grey matter in their brains—this is the matter where all of the nerves and decision-making happens, so this is kind of a big deal.

Coffee

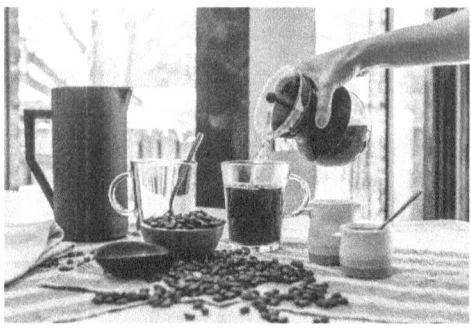

In moderation, coffee is great for you! This does not mean that you should go out and drink a Venti mocha every day. However — the sugar in that mocha can actually do you more harm than good. However, straight coffee is primarily caffeine and antioxidants.

Both of these are great for the brain. Caffeine keeps you awake longer, alert more, and makes you feel better. It has been shown that these boosts from caffeine have also boosted concentration as well.

Long-term coffee usage has also been found to be related to lessened risk of Alzheimer's and Parkinson's, quite possibly thanks to all of the antioxidants contained within it.

Broccoli

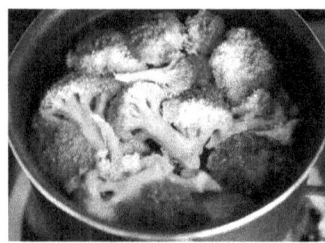

This is another plant filled with powerful antioxidants. However, broccoli also brings with it vitamin K, which is critical for the use of sphingolipids, which are the fats that the brain uses.

Those who regularly consume vitamin K tend to show that they have better functional memories than those who have less, making this an important link to consider.

Blueberries

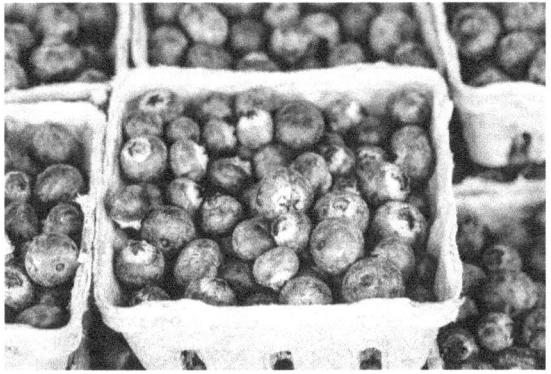

Again, you see high concentrations of antioxidants in blueberries. These are present in the anthocyanins, which give the dark color that people associate with the berries to begin with.
They have anti-inflammatory and antioxidant properties, and both of these help defend the brain and keep it healthy.

Turmeric

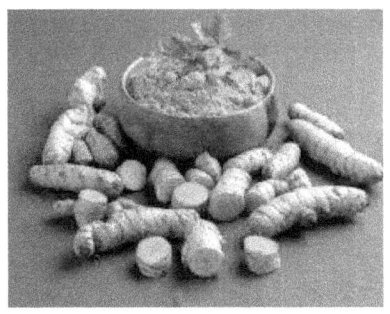

This spice is commonly associated with curry powder and Indian food, and is a delicious addition to your food. It is anti-inflammatory and has plenty of antioxidant effects, and thanks to Curcumin, the main compound found in turmeric, it is able to cross the blood-brain barrier, allowing for a much more direct influence.
This means that it can help with memory, having been shown to benefit those suffering from
Alzheimer's. It has also been shown to ease depression and help with the growth of brain cells thanks to the boost in the growth hormone it creates.

Pumpkin seeds

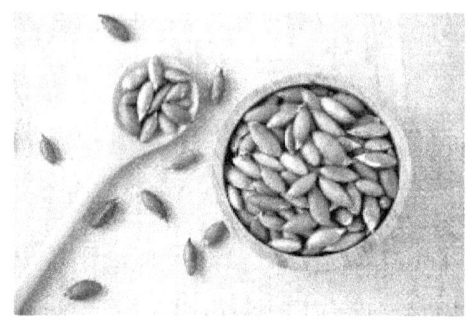

Once again, rich in antioxidants, pumpkin seeds also bring with them several other nutrients as well, such as zinc, magnesium, copper, and iron. Your brain needs all of these to facilitate growth, development, and function, and without enough, you may find that you struggle with brain fog.

Eggs

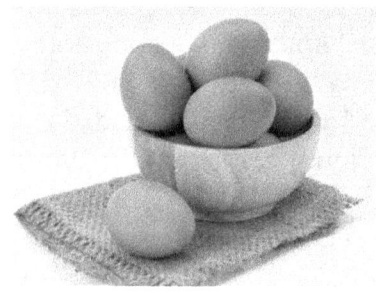

Eggs provide plenty of nutrients that are necessary for healthy brain development, such as B6, B12, and folate. All of these are necessary for your brain to function well. Eggs also bring with them choline, a nutrient that is responsible for the creation of acetylcholine, which is used heavily in both memory formation and mood regulation. Egg yolks, in particular, have a quarter of your necessary choline for the day, making them one of the most potently concentrated foods for choline.

Physical Exercises for the Brain

Exercise is also absolutely essential if you want to have good brain health. Hitting the gym is actually fantastic to make sure that your brain is functioning properly. This is why so many people with depression and anxiety are told to get up and get moving—it helps! In particular, you will see the most boost in the brain if you add aerobic exercise to your daily routine.

This does not mean that you have to go off and begin working out like your life depends upon it—even just 20 minutes a day is going to show you a noticeable improvement in brain function for most people.

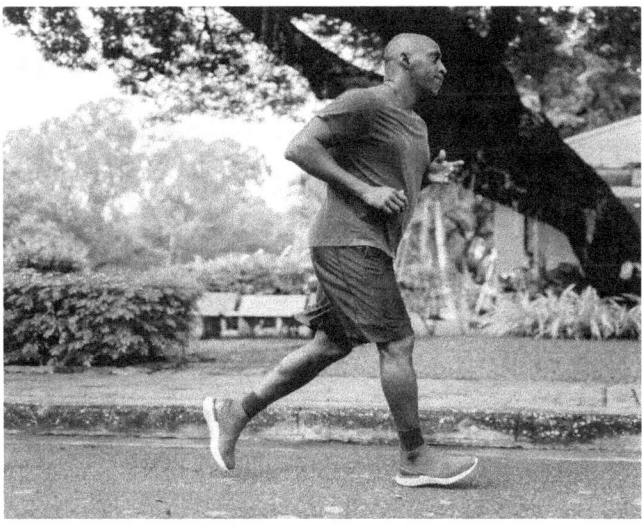

This happens because of the effect that exercise has on the body as a whole. When you exercise, your heart rate increases.

This means that more blood is pumped throughout your body, and therefore to your brain. With more oxygen available in the brain, the brain can think and act with more clarity and efficiency.

Beyond just that, however, when you exercise, you cause all sorts of hormones to flood your body. These hormones allow for your body to work on repairing itself.

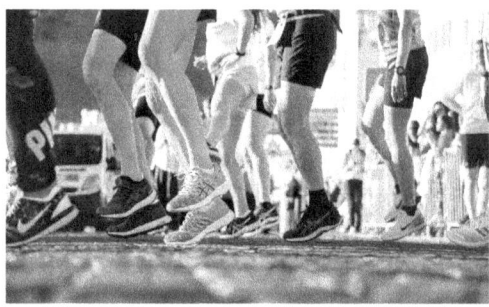

With this, the brain is also able to begin stimulating new growth. It is able to actively improve the connections between cells, reinforcing those synapses, and making sure that the brain is functioning at optimal levels.

Think for a moment about runner's highs—people who run say they feel like they get a high when they are running.

This is for a good reason—when you run, you drop stress hormones, and that means that the hippocampus is able to function better. It is able to grow more.

The hippocampus, in particular, is the part of your brain that is responsible for memory making so it becomes an important part to boost the function of if you are looking to train your brain.

When you want to exercise for your brain, there are a few things to keep in mind to really optimize the effects.

Of course, these are general guidelines, and ultimately, your body is going to see improvements in function even with less exercise added into the daily routine, so do what you can.

If what you can do is everything within these suggestions, then great! If not, don't sweat it—well, get out and sweat, but do not worry about it too much.

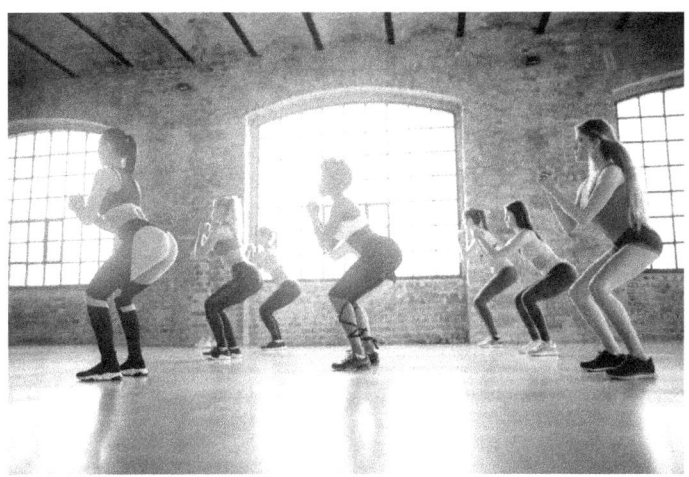

- **If it is good for your heart, it will be just as good for your brain:**
  When you work your heart, you send more blood to the brain, which means the brain gets more energy

- **Aerobic exercise is best:**
  This will allow for brain function to improve as well as allowing for the healing of other brain cells within the body already that are damaged

- **Aim to exercise in the morning:**

    When you exercise specifically in the morning, you will find that your brain activity rises. You will set up for the day to actively retain new information, you will feel less stressed out as you start your day, and you will find that you respond better to any stress that arises.

- **Coordination-based aerobics are preferred:**

    When you do something that not only requires you to be incredibly active but also quite coordinated, you are making your brain work out more with your heart at the same time. Dance classes or other high-energy exercises with coordination will be your best bet for seeing the most improvement.

- **If you are short on time, go for circuit workouts:**

    These are workouts where you are keeping your heart rate high but also constantly changing what you are doing. This requires your brain to be on high alert, adapting with you as you go. When you stop and compare what your brain has to do if you are mindlessly running on a treadmill versus what you are doing if you are switching from running to hopping to doing stairs, or anything else in your circuit, you will start to see the importance of changing it up constantly. Your brain is kept busier, and a busy brain is a healthy brain.

- **If you are currently exhausted, try a quick cardio exercise:**

    You do not have to run to the gym just because you are tired. However, stopping and doing a few rounds of jumping jacks, quite possibly with a coffee, will largely improve your function, at least temporarily. If you have that deadline looming and you are feeling exhausted, this may be the best bet for you.

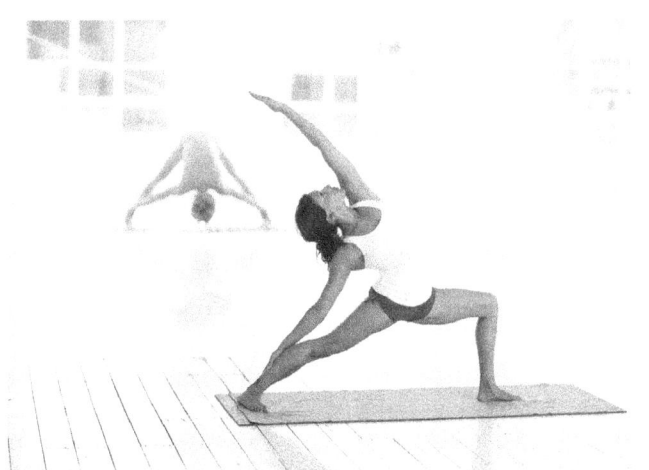

Overall, any exercise is good for you, whether it is incredibly active or it is slower. Not everyone can exercise quite so aerobically, and that is okay!

Just keeping yourself busy and moving your body is still good for you, and you will still see an improvement in how you feel, even if you add in low-impact exercises, such as swimming, or if you stick to cycling at home or even just going for a daily walk.

What matters most is that you get up and get moving. Your body, and your brain, will thank you for it.

Conclusion

Congratulations! You have made it to the end of Brain Training! It has been quite a journey, and hopefully, it has been useful to you in some capacity.

People these days get stuck in a brain fog and feel like that is just how they have to live.

People may assume that they are not smart because they cannot do mental math or because they struggle to remember things.

However, remember, your intelligence and your mental abilities are both things that you can actively and deliberately change.

Your brain is just like any other muscle in your body—while it is not actually a muscle, it still requires the same sort of upkeep as a muscle.

Left without any stimulation or practice, your brain will begin to prune connections. This is why you struggle to remember any of the Spanish you learned in middle school, or why you may feel like you cannot possibly recall how to balance equations in Chemistry after having been great at it before.

If you do not practice and use the information that your brain is storing, it will forget it, It will prune those synapses to make space for new ones, and this means that you are actively going to lose information that you worked so hard to remember.

Treat your brain like any other muscle in your body—in fact, treat it like the most important muscle in your body, as this is what is responsible for making you who you are. If you want to boost those memory making abilities, then you need to use them on a regular basis.

Train your brain. Teach yourself new things. Make it a point to learn a new instrument or how to paint or speak a new language.
Your brain loves to learn thing—that is exactly what it is meant to do, and without a constant influx of things to do, your brain will start to weaken.

From here, you are probably going to be best served by making sure that you are actively engaging your brain on a regular basis.
Make sure that you are actively spending time training it—play mental games. Learn to speed read. Do anything that forces your brain to work.
Over time, you will find that your ability to think quickly and on your feet improves.
You will find that you are able to better regulate yourself. You will find that you are able to remember things far more than you were before.
You will find that, above all, you are happier.
You are no longer looking through life in a fog, and instead are actively engaging yourself, your mind, and learning.
You are doing what you were meant to do, and that will be satisfying.

As this book comes to a close, do not forget that you should always be willing to try new things.
Do not forget the benefit that novelty and a break in fluency bring to your brain.
Remember just how much you are capable of and do not let you convince yourself otherwise.
You can train your brain.
You can read faster.
You can remember more.
You do so much more than you think that you can.
All you need to do is try, and try some more.
Keep with it, and you will succeed!

Finally, if you have found this book to be useful in any capacity, please head over to Amazon to leave a review! Your feedback is appreciated and valued, and will help in the development of further books.

Thank you so much for taking this journey with this book in your hand, and good luck as you put these techniques to good use!

Did this book help you in some way? If so, I'd love to hear about it. Honest reviews help readers find the right book for their needs."

www.ingramcontent.com/pod-product-compliance
Lightning Source LLC
Chambersburg PA
CBHW071413210526
45465CB00001B/364